THE FUNCTIONAL STRENGTH TRAINING

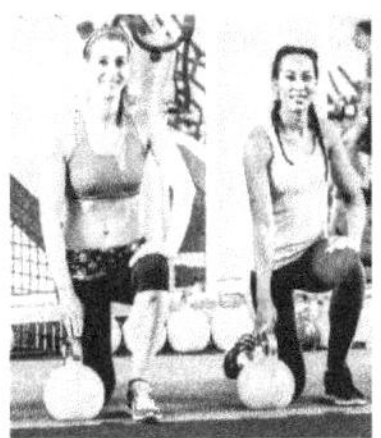

The Complete guide to building muscle for anatomy energy to stay healthy and lose weight

Jay A. Beams

ABOUT AUTHOR

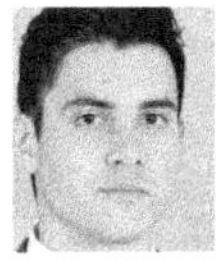 Jay A. Beams, a seasoned author and fitness virtuoso dedicated to sculpting not just bodies, but transforming lives. With a passion for training and a pen that wields inspiration, Jay has become a guiding force in the realm of health and fitness. His literary endeavors serve as a roadmap for countless individuals, navigating them towards the pinnacle of their well-being. Through the pages of his books,Beams doesn't just share knowledge; he sparks a revolution, empowering readers to conquer their fitness goals and embrace a healthier, more vibrant life.

Table of contents

Introduction

Enter a world where strength is a testament to the functionality of every fiber in your body rather than merely a measurement of muscle. We reveal the techniques that transcend the traditional in this ground-breaking manual on functional strength training, reframing power as a harmonious union of the mind and body. Prepare yourself for a life-changing experience where turning each page will bring you one step closer to realizing your own potential. This book is more than simply a book; it's your key to an extraordinary world of power, calling to those who desire a complete transformation of their being as opposed to merely physical strength. Greetings from the strength training of the future.

Where power and utility converge in the world of fitness, a life-changing adventure awaits those who are willing to take it on. Greetings from a universe where all movements are evidence of inner strength. In "Functional Strength Training," get ready to discover a comprehensive approach to wellness in addition to physical capability. This is a manual for creating a strong physique and an endlessly energetic existence, not just a book. Come along with me as one functional rep at a time, we redefine strength.

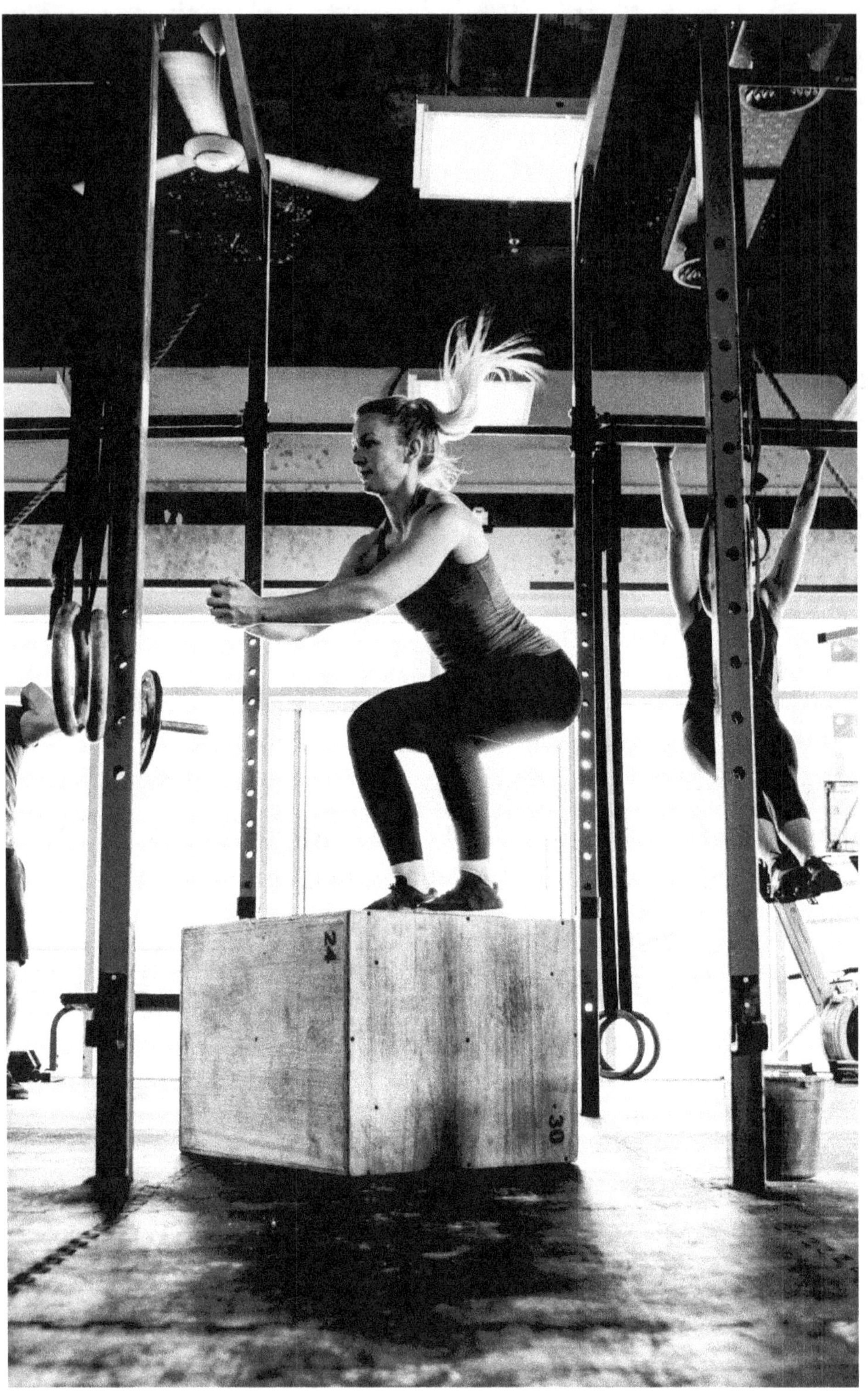

Chapter 1

What Functional Strength Training Is For

Functional strength training (FST): what is it exactly? "Training that attempts to mimic the specific physiological demands of real-life activities" is the definition of functional strength training. It simply means using the body in the manner for which it was designed. There's a chance that this kind of instruction will simplify daily duties. Minimize the chance of injury. Boost your standard of living.

Rather than concentrating on building a single muscle or group of muscles, functional strength training aims to strengthen many muscle groups and joints simultaneously.

FITNESS FOR WHOM CAN FUNCTIONAL STRENGTH TRAINING BENEFIT? In summary, everybody can benefit from functional strength training. It is a great form of exercise that is good for people of all ages. Every fitness level Before beginning a strength training program, always get in touch with a doctor or a certified fitness trainer, especially if you don't exercise frequently. In addition, beginners should limit their use of functional strength training to their own body weight. You can use heavier weights or resistance bands to boost resistance as your strength grows.

 Senior Citizens' Useful Strength Training If used in conjunction with other comprehensive programs to help older adults improve their balance, functional strength training may be highly beneficial. Become more agile. It is necessary to strengthen your muscles. Cut down on the likelihood of falling. Functional Strength Training for Athletes In addition, functional strength training is beneficial for athletes getting ready to compete in a particular sport. This is so that functional strength training programs may be tailored to the unique motions of each athlete.

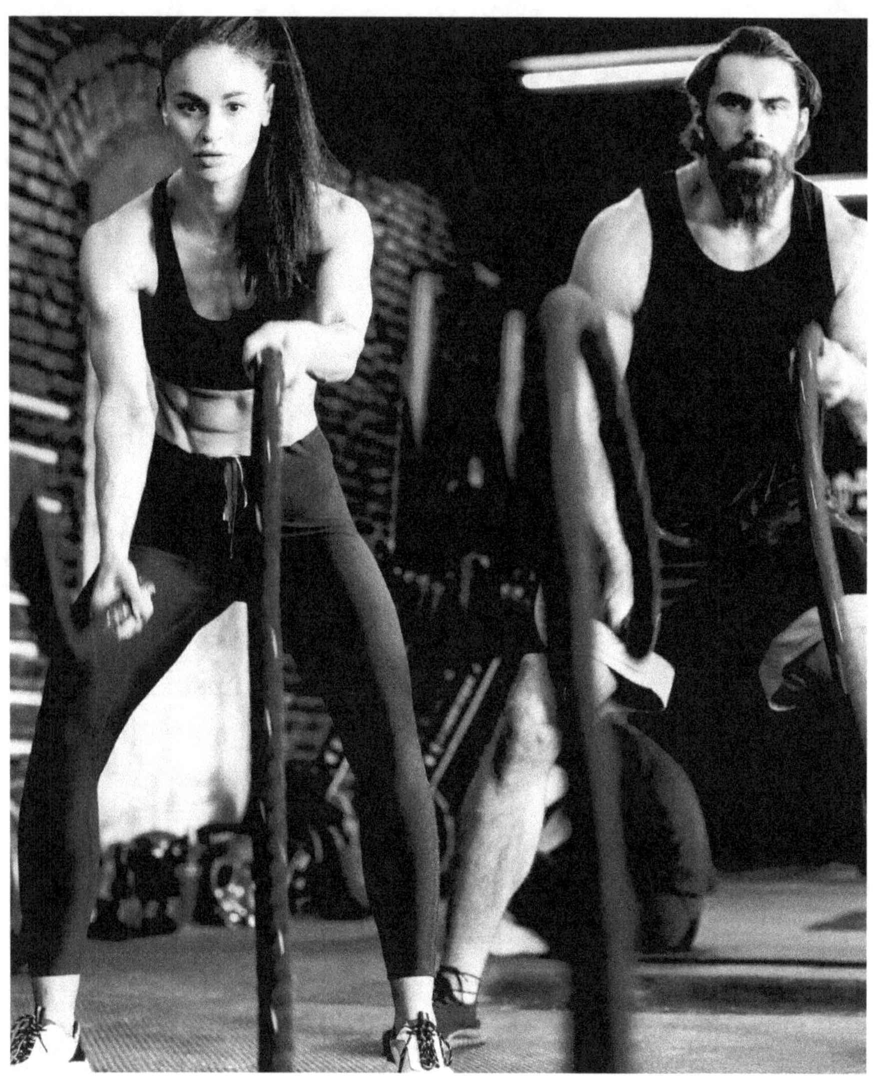

For instance, functional strength training for tennis players will seem different from that of triathletes. The Goal of Functional Strength Training Exercises Numerous joints and muscles are used during functional activities. It's a great way to activate and enliven your entire body at once. For example, a functional workout can simultaneously target the elbows, shoulders, hips, knees, and ankles. Imagine walking into a typical gym. You can head to the dumbbell racks if you wish to engage in some strength training.

As an alternative, you might bench press a barbell to start. But think about your daily life. Is your daily routine something like curling a 15-pound dumbbell or benching a bar? Perhaps not. "Carrying barbells and dumbbells around is not how the body was designed to be used." Fitness instructors at Motion O.C. recommend functional exercises that align the body's natural motions." Functional fitness is the absence of aimlessness.

MINDLESS MOVEMENT: WHAT DOES IT MEAN? Think about the following motions: Pull-Push Squat Twist Lunge These are the movements required to carry out the daily duties you perform. As examples, consider: Going for a walk Getting out of a chair Trying to reach for something on a shelf, or getting on your hands and knees to tie your shoes glancing back to see what's behind you while moving big objects across rooms You don't consider your movements when engaging in such activities. All you have to do is execute them. You're traveling in circles.

Let's examine this one more time. Think about how kids move. Kids wander around aimlessly. Children are not "in their heads" when they run, leap, play, and pick up objects. They're not thinking about doing such a thing. The idea of moving aimlessly, or organically, is crucial to functional strength training. However, we recognize that while the goal is to move mindlessly, it may not always be easy to figure out how to do so in the gym. The key is that creating a functional exercise program doesn't have to be difficult. Let In Motion O.C. take care of it. Our fitness instructors are masters at designing effective strength-training workout plans. They will create a program to assist you become stronger and more mobile so you may live a more efficient and pain-free life. How often should one perform exercises involving functional strength training? You can perform functional strength training programs on a daily basis without worrying about damage because functional movements mimic everyday chores. You should try to perform these exercises two or three times a week.

You don't have to drag yourself to the gym on a daily basis, though. Tools for Strengthening Your Function Barbells and other equipment are not required. What then are the prerequisites for functional strength training? Simplicity is essential when it comes to practical strength training equipment. Most functional exercises use your own body weight as resistance. This implies that you can perform these workouts at home or at a park, depending on your preference. Exercises that involve more than just body weight include: Weights Kettlebells Balls for medicine Resistance bands bars that chin up Functional Strength Training Has Six Benefits What makes exercising with function in mind then? There are various benefits to this type of strength training. They are listed in the following order: delaying the start of muscle atrophy associated with aging Agility and coordination are enhanced.

The balance is now better. enhances core strength lessens the chance of injury The pain lessens as you gain strength.

#1: MILD THE IMPACT OF MUSCLE ATROPHY RELATED TO AGE Loss of muscle mass is known as muscular atrophy. Along with this loss of muscle mass comes a loss of strength. The medical name for this is sarcopenia. After middle age, adults lose 3% of their muscle mass year. Over time, this could become increasingly difficult to do everyday tasks. Getting more exercise is the best way to prevent muscle loss. This is due to the fact that inactivity is one of the main causes of muscle loss in addition to aging. It's a common saying to "use it or lose it." Muscle atrophy has been shown to be considerably reduced and even reversed by functional strength training.

#2 ADVANTAGES: AGILITY AND COORDINATION According to one definition, coordination is "the ability to use different parts of one's body together smoothly and efficiently." Meanwhile, "the ability to move quickly and easily" is the definition of agility. Leaping, squatting, lunging, and other functional strength training exercises can improve your coordination and agility.

#3: IMPROVES BALANCE When doing functional strength training, compound motions are employed. These challenging exercises help you improve balance. Everyone benefits from this, but seniors especially so because improved balance lowers the risk of falling.

#4: Fortifies the Center You might immediately think of your abdominal muscles when you think about core strengthening. Your core, nevertheless, is far more than that. As a matter of fact, your core consists of as many as thirty-five different muscle groups that run from your chest to your hips. A good core is necessary for most full-body exercises. Think of your body as a building. A strong foundation is necessary for a structure's protection and support. The foundation of your body is your core. If you're hurt or uncomfortable, you probably don't have a solid base.

Strength training that is functional might be helpful here. Activating many muscle groups simultaneously enhances core stability. A well-supported body and a stronger core help one avoid pain when performing daily tasks.

#5: LOWERS THE RISK OF INJURY Functional strength training exercises maintain your joints stable and active. While increasing your functional strength and mobility increases your body's stress level, it also reduces your risk of injury. Here are a few instances of this kind: Lowering the chance of knee pain and injury, squats improve knee strength and mobility. Planks assist lessen lower back pain and damage by strengthening the core. Exercise bikes are a great way to warm up before strength training because, let's face it, you rode them when you were younger.

 #6: As you become stronger, your pain levels decrease. Do you have an injury or are you in chronic pain? Don't let that stop you from working out. Don't sacrifice going to the park or the gym for your sofa. While recovering from an injury, rest is essential. However, with the correct guidance from a physical therapist or certified fitness coach, functional strength training may also help. Making your daily motions pain-free is the aim of functional fitness.

Gaining strength will improve the efficiency of your body's movements. Your degree of pain will consequently decrease.

Benefits and Importance

Why are functional fitness benefits so great? Anybody can benefit from functional fitness programs, regardless of age, fitness level, prior exercise experience, or available training time.

Functional training programs may help with muscular growth, aerobic capability, calorie burning, and muscle definition. Simply moving—especially in several directions, at different speeds, and with a variety of exercise equipment to activate every muscle in the body—is the fundamental element of a functional training session. Find out the eight unique benefits of functional training regimens by reading on.

1. Better Movement Patterns: Movement is innate to the human body. Functional training exercises focus more on movement patterns than on discrete muscle actions. Because of its unique design, the human body functions best when it is moving straight ahead with both feet planted on the ground. Human movement can be categorized into patterns like the hinge, squat, lunge, pull, and push movements that occur both overhead and towards the front of the body, as well as rotation. The Nautilus HumanSport cable strength-training equipment allow users to perform all movement patterns from a standing position, maximizing the advantages of their workouts.

2. Enhanced Movement Efficiency: To help players reach their maximum potential in their sport, functional strength training methods are used. To assist their players compete better, a lot of strength and conditioning instructors base their exercise programs on movement patterns. Coach Mike Boyle, who owns Mike Boyle Strength and Conditioning outside of Boston, Massachusetts, and is the author of New Functional Training for Sports, has been using this system with his athletes for many years. Many of these athletes participate at the highest levels of collegiate and professional sports. "Functional training is best characterized by exercises done with the feet in contact with the ground and, with few exceptions, without the aid of machines," says Boyle. Since they require users to do the lifts while

standing, many barbell workouts done on a Throwdown XTC Rig with a landmine attachment are very functional under this criteria.

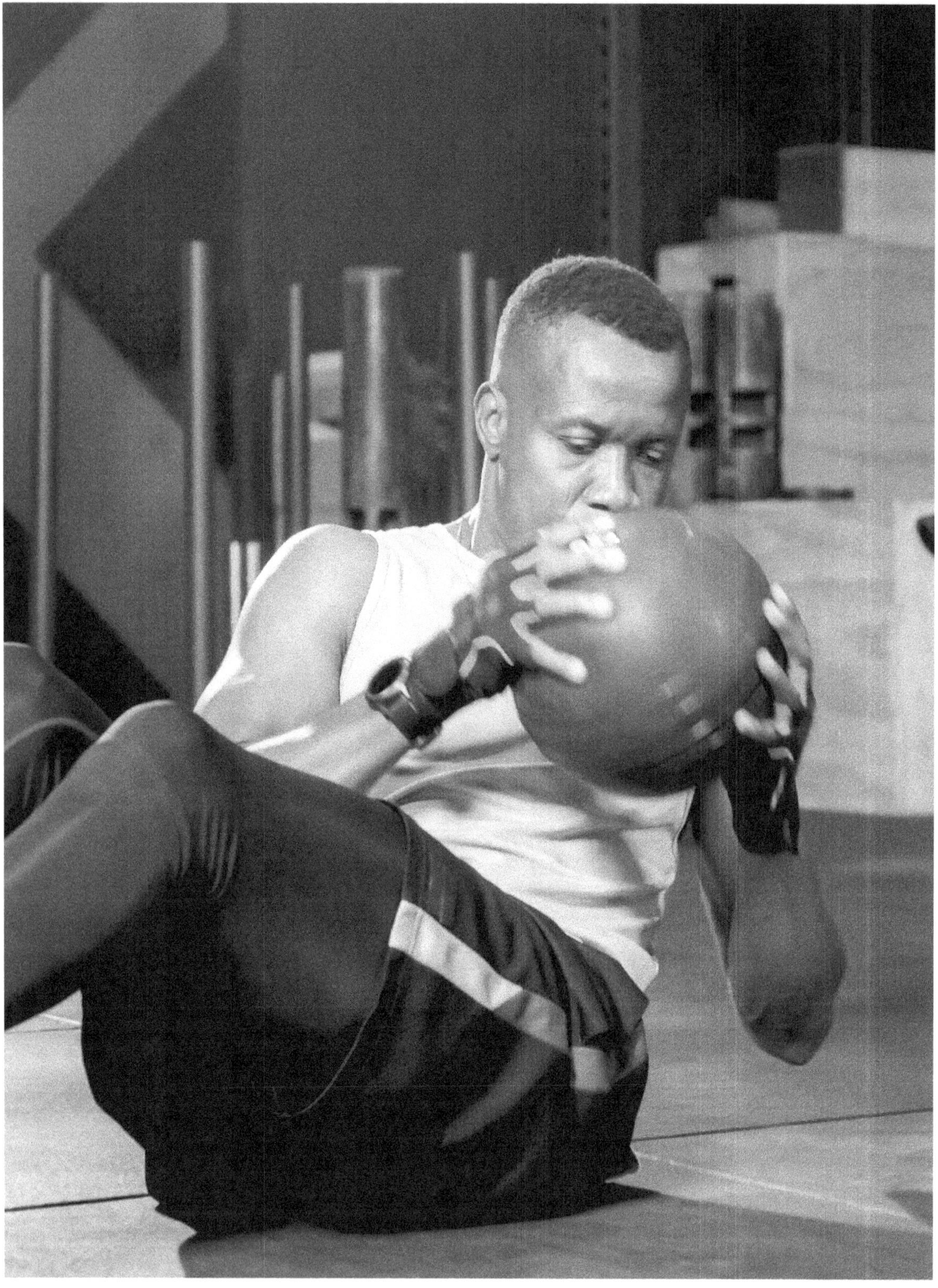

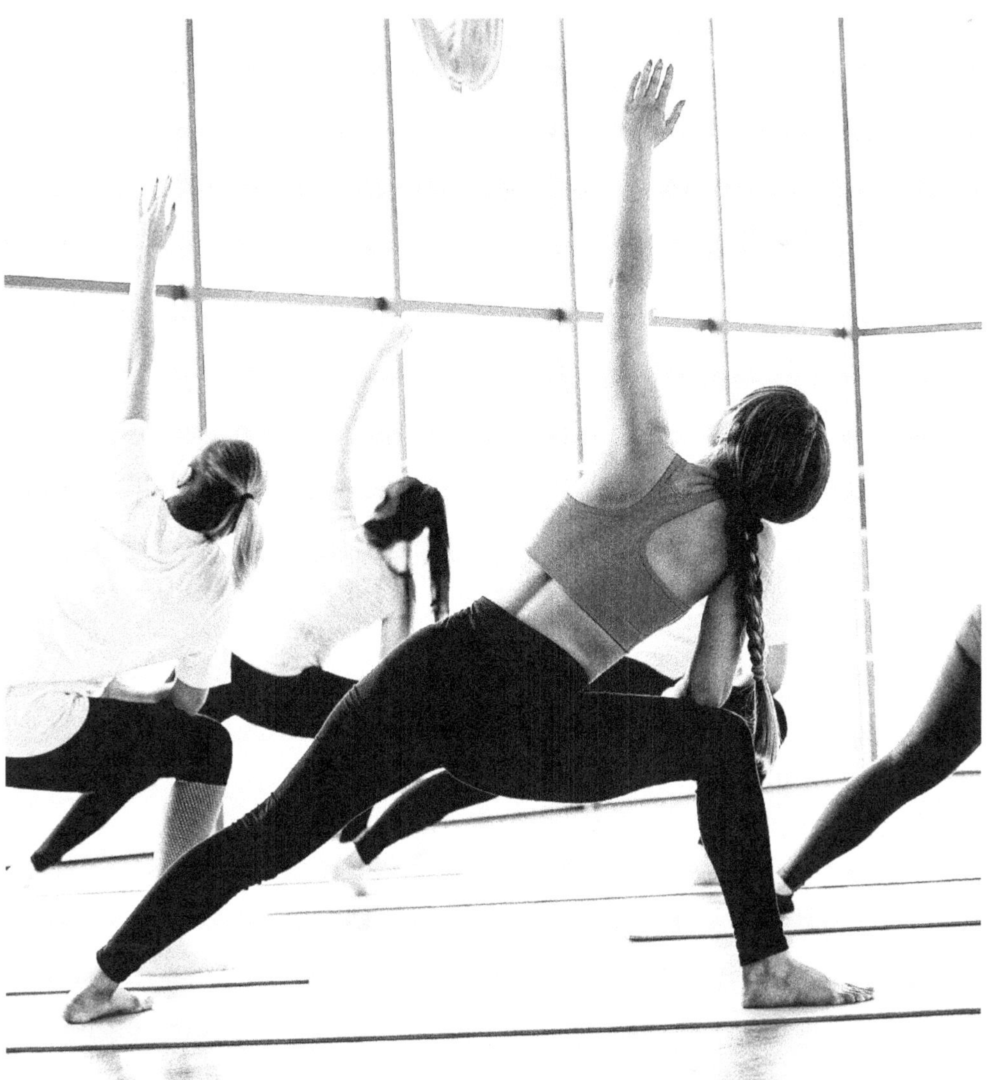

3. Improved Physical appearance: By working many muscular groups simultaneously, functional training can help achieve a leaner, more athletic appearance. Due to their usage of their entire body, many athletes and dancers have amazing physique. It may be possible for users to get the same lean, muscular appearance as people who are paid to move for a living by using the Nautilus HumanSport equipment for functional, movement-based exercises.

4. Enhanced Coordination and Mobility: Functional training exercises can help reduce the risk of injury by improving overall coordination and mobility. The capacity to regulate movement throughout a full range of motion is known as mobility. Several integrated movement patterns, like squats and pushing and pulling while standing, can enhance joint mobility while simultaneously enhancing

overall muscle coordination. This is because when muscles on one side of a joint shorten, muscles on the other side lengthen. Using the Olympic bar station on the Throwdown XTC Rig for a bent-over row emphasizes the pulling pattern, which can enhance shoulder range-of-motion, particularly with a palms-up grip, and coordination between all the deep core and lower body muscles that stabilize the body.

5. Increased Calorie Burn: Functional training has the potential to increase calorie burn in comparison to traditional strength training. The body uses about five calories of energy to ingest one liter of oxygen. You burn more calories and utilize more oxygen when you exercise more muscles. Think about it: standing squat-to-row on a cable machine like the Nautilus HumanSport Freedom Trainer or sitting rowing on a bench will use more muscles?

6. Enhanced Aerobic Capacity: Functional cardio training is another name for High-Intensity Interval Training (HIIT). Using a StairMaster HIIT Rower or HIIT Bike, a 4-minute Tabata routine consists of 8 rounds, each lasting 20 seconds at maximum exertion. The results of a 4-minute Tabata cycle and a 30-minute treadmill run were examined in a recent study. While the 30-minute group ran at a moderate level of exertion for a total of 90 minutes per week, the Tabata interval group engaged in high-intensity interval training (HIIT) for 12 minutes each week. At the end of the study, the Tabata group outperformed the 30-minute treadmill group in terms of both aerobic capacity and time to fatigue.

7. Enhanced Lean Muscle Mass: HIIT on a StairMaster HIIT Rower combined with explosive medicine ball throws or heavy barbell lifts performed on the Throwdown XTC Rig as part of a functional training program may help active seniors preserve their strength and lean muscle mass well into old age. Muscle fibers are 'use-it-or-lose-it' materials. Strength and definition-producing type II muscle fibers may atrophy if they are not used during exercise. This would lead to a loss of strength and definition. Type II muscle fibers, which are frequently underutilized in lower-intensity training routines, are targeted and engaged by high-intensity activities. Aging and high-intensity training are both challenging. People can maintain their strength and fitness far into their senior years by

following an exercise program that is specifically intended to help mitigate the effects of aging.

8. Class Design Ease: Small group training sessions on the Nautilus HumanSport line or the Throwdown XTC Rig may offer the benefits of functional training while yet adhering to the laws of social distancing. The Throwdown XTC Rigs allow multiple users to interact without being too close to one another by arranging the stations. It is possible to arrange the Nautilus HumanSport equipment to allow for adequate isolation. The human body is capable of carrying out a wide range of tasks when used properly.

It takes a variety of varied motions in a training program to effectively activate and excite muscles. Exercise programs can be created using equipment like the Nautilus HumanSport, Throwdown XTC Rig, or StairMaster HIIT circuit. This equipment can be placed with the right spacing to produce highly functional and effective workouts, as well as to push the body in a variety of ways.

Comprehending Functional Strength

Benefits of Functional Strength Training for True Strength: The goal of functional strength training is to enhance general strength, flexibility, and athletic performance by concentrating on resistance exercises that mimic everyday activities.

Functional strength training (FST): what is it exactly? Functional strength training teaches your body to move correctly during everyday tasks including standing, sitting, climbing stairs, and lifting large objects. These exercises increase overall strength levels when resistance is introduced, which makes daily tasks easier to do. Increasing resistance also enables you to link strength training to actual performance motions, which enables you to apply your gym work to everyday tasks, athletic events, or recreational pursuits. Exercises for functional strength training involve multi-joint motions that work multiple muscle groups simultaneously; these types of exercises are sometimes called compound exercises. Along with strength, balance, coordination, and stability are also promoted by this type of training.

You can utilize a variety of resistance tools and equipment to change the intensity of the workout. Begin with bodyweight squats and work your way up to weighted barbell squats. You can also use bands, medicine balls, or suspension trainers to increase the resistance. Your learning curve might not be as steep as you think because you may already be familiar with squats, push-ups, pull-ups, and deadlifts! If you're not familiar with this phrase, don't worry.
 Remain motivated and stick to your fitness objectives.

Benefits of Functional Strength Training: The benefits of functional strength training are easily perceived and experienced. In fact, incorporating this training methodology throughout your entire program may assist improve your general level of fitness, athletic ability, risk of injury, and ability to exercise more effectively. Enhanced overall fitness: By simultaneously stimulating multiple joints, functional strength training—especially complex exercises—can improve movement ability and dynamic balance. Additionally, it enhances muscle flexibility, mobility, and coordination—all of which lead to an improvement in general fitness and quality of life. Enhanced Athletic Performance: A major goal of functional strength training is to get your body ready for the everyday movements required for optimal athletic performance. If you're an athlete, you may tailor functional strength training to the demands of your particular sport by focusing on the muscle groups and movements that are essential for optimal performance.

Athletes' power, balance, agility, speed, and muscle strength may all be enhanced via functional training. Prevention and Treatment of Injuries: Including functional strength training exercises for all major muscle groups promotes balanced muscular growth, which may help prevent musculoskeletal disorders brought on by imbalanced muscle tissue. It also helps to prevent conditions related to the low back. More effective workouts: Functional strength training, at its core, aims to work many muscle groups simultaneously, as opposed to working each area independently. By using a comprehensive strategy, you may workout more efficiently and utilize your time, strength, energy, and rest periods to the fullest. Fundamentals of Functional Strength Training: Multi-joint exercises and intricate functional movement patterns incorporating many muscle groups, like the lunge, pull-ups, push-ups, loaded carries, squat, and deadlift, are instances of functional strength training. To achieve overall balance and functional fitness, you will focus on full-body exercises while designing a functional strength training program, taking care not to overemphasize some muscle groups while neglecting others.

With this type of training, your body can work as a whole instead of as separate parts. You can also use it to target movements that are crucial for daily living, activities, and athletic performance. The progressive overload idea, which calls for gradually increasing intensity, resistance, or complexity to keep the muscles challenged and encourage development, strength, power, and improvement, is also the foundation of functional strength training.

A fundamental idea of functional strength training is the capacity to perform workouts in the sagittal, frontal, and transverse planes of motion. Joint motions that are possible in each plane include flexion, extension, abduction, adduction, rotation, dorsiflexion, plantarflexion, elevation, depression, inversion, eversion, pronation, supination, horizontal flexion, and horizontal extension.

Incorporating functional strength training exercises into fitness regimens that focus on all three planes of motion ensures that your body trains as it does in real life. This approach also helps to create a well-rounded routine. Exercises for Functional Strength: Common movement patterns including hinging, squatting, pushing, pulling, and rotating are frequently modeled by multi-joint motions used in functional strength training exercises.

These fundamental functional strength training methods can be included into your exercise regimen. Squats and Their Variations: The squat is a fundamental lower body action pattern. All of the major muscles in the lower body, including the quadriceps, hamstrings, gluteus maximus, gluteus minimus, gluteus medius, adductors, hip flexors, and calves, are worked throughout this dynamic exercise. Your core muscles, especially the rectus abdominis, transverse abdominis, obliques, and erector spinae, are crucial for proper movement execution even if your legs and glutes will do most of the heavy lifting. Additionally—the best part? You can choose from a variety of squat variations, so you should never get bored performing this crucial functional strength training exercise! To make the move more challenging, you can also use a variety of tools. A barbell or dumbbell is the most common tool used to increase the resistance in a squat. But you may also use resistance bands, kettlebells, TRX suspension trainers, or a Smith machine. Exercises and variations for the squat include the front, back, ply, goblet, split, split squat in Bulgaria, pistol squats, box squats, and squat jump variations on deadlifts. The deadlift exercise requires a hip flexion.

When picking something up off the floor, for example, this practical movement pattern is employed. The gluteus maximus, hamstrings, and lower back are worked during deadlifts. They also work a variety of upper-body muscles because they require lifting weight off the ground. You might experience low back pain and other postural issues if you have back weakness. This is especially true for people who sit for extended periods of time. The good news is that you may strengthen these crucial posterior muscles by performing a proper deadlift.

Similar to the squat, the deadlift can be done with a range of resistance equipment. The majority of deadlift workouts use dumbbells, hex bars, trap bars, kettlebells, and barbells. You can choose from the following deadlift exercises and variations: push-ups and their variations, traditional deadlift, deadlift in Romania, deadlift sumo, deadlift on one leg alone, and deadlift with stiff-legged legs.

There are few exercises that are as timeless as the push-up. In this functional strength training exercise, your upper and lower body muscles must cooperate to move your body in both directions—that is, toward and away from the ground. Your lower body and core muscles will provide stability and support, but your chest, shoulders, and triceps will be doing the bulk of the lifting. One great thing about push-ups as an exercise is that they don't require any special equipment. On the other hand, using tools like a weight bench, suspension trainer, stability ball, or push-up bars are examples of additional adjustments.

Exercises and variations of push-ups include: standard push-ups performed with a tight grip; push-ups performed with only one arm; push-ups performed on bent knees; push-ups performed on an incline or decline using a bench; push-ups performed with claps; push-ups performed in a diamond shape; and push-ups performed with a TRX pull-up and its variations. You should feel your core muscles attempting to maintain your torso if you perform these exercises correctly. You can perform a pull-up using a pull-up bar or a weight-assisted equipment called a Gravitron if you have access to a gym. By lowering the amount of weight you must lift, a banded pull-up can help simplify the exercise. There are several variations and exercises for pull-ups, such as the standard pull-up, the broad grip pull-up, the tight grip pull-up, the reverse pull-up, banded pull-ups with assistance, the Gravitron lift-up, planks, and core exercises. Exercises involving planks and the core help to improve balance, stability, and overall functional fitness. The muscles in your abdomen, lower back, pelvis, and hips are your "core" muscles.

They work similarly to an internal weight belt in that they reduce the risk of injury and improve overall body control by providing stability and support to your pelvis and spine during dynamic movements. Additionally, a strong core enhances performance in a range of physical activities, including bodyweight exercises, weightlifting, and athletics. Planks and other core exercises are excellent compound movements for functional training since they work the muscles of the shoulders, arms, legs, and glutes in addition to the core. Moreover, the majority of exercises only require your bodyweight as resistance! Planks and core exercises consist of the following: forearm planks; side planks followed by a shoulder tap; Deadbug Farmer's stroll; Canine Bird Pallof press (requires cable machine); How to Start Functional Strength Training It's easy to start functional strength training once you know the correct techniques.

Please make sure you obtain permission before doing anything if you need it from your physician or another medical professional. Once the all clear is given, it's a good idea to speak with a physical therapist or personal trainer to assess your current level of fitness and work together to create a program that meets your needs. They might also help you set goals relating to your fitness, provide you guidance on how to go forward safely, and show you how to include functional strength training into your whole exercise program. assessing existing fitness level See a qualified personal trainer, strength and conditioning coach, or physical therapist to ascertain your current fitness level prior to starting a functional strength training program.

To ensure that the exercises you choose are appropriate for your ability level, they could put you through a range of fitness tests. Establishing Goals and Designing a Program: An effective strength training regimen should include exercises that maximize muscle strength and endurance, target specific muscle groups, lessen muscle imbalances, increase mobility and coordination, and improve athletic performance. Core functional motions such as squat, lunge, hinge, push, pull, rotation, and gait are examples of movements that are used in daily activities. Range of motion, coordination, movement speed, and various muscular contraction types, such as concentric, eccentric, and isometric, should all be the focus of functional strength training exercises. Additionally, you want to select functional strength training exercises that are similar to the skill, activity, or movement that you hope to improve. When designing a program, the duration and number of days of instruction are crucial components to take into account.

The Physical Activity Guidelines for Americans, which advise people to perform moderate-to-intense muscle-strengthening exercises involving all major muscle groups two or more days a week, are a great source of information about how often to exercise. This is on top of 150 to 300 minutes a week of moderate-intensity aerobic or cardiovascular exercise or 75 to 150 minutes a week of evenly spaced out vigorous-intensity physical activity. For optimal strength growth and top performance, you can vary your training stimulus with Gradual Progression and Intensification Periodization. Depending on your goals, a periodized program's volume and intensity will change. For instance, a lot of programs begin with larger volumes and lower intensities and progress to exercises with intermediate volumes and intensities before moving on to exercises with lower volumes and intensities. Including Functional Strength Training in Your Exercise Program: Including functional strength training into an existing exercise program is one of the many advantages of this approach.

One way to get started with this training method if you're new to it is to incorporate some simple functional strength training exercises into your warm-up, like squats or lunges. You may also try switching up traditional strength training exercises like seated leg presses and biceps curls with functional ones like banded pull-ups and kettlebell squats. Because full-body exercises are a common part of functional strength training, you should plan proper recuperation days. To allow for three to four training days per week, it is a good idea to take one day off in between workouts.

Exercises that require endurance, sports, or moderate-to-high-intensity cardio should be included in your fitness program; otherwise, you might want to limit your full-body functional strength training sessions to two or three days per week. Gyms and fitness centers are filled with equipment for functional strength training exercises. Many of these pieces of gear are perfect for beginners or those who want extra support in one or more body areas. They can also be added to other sports-specific routines or functional strength training. Free weights demand you to use your primary movers and stabilizer muscles to control the weight throughout its complete range of motion, while resistance machines offer stabilization and have a predetermined pattern of action. These are some common resistance tools and equipment that can be used when performing functional strength training exercises, though this is not an exhaustive list: bodyweight dumbbells, barbells, kettlebells, resistance bands, suspension shoes, bars for chin-ups, medical balls, weighted bags, and common mistakes made when performing functional strength training exercises.

Although functional strength training has many potential benefits, there are a few common mistakes people make when engaging in it. Here are some things to keep in mind when working out: Skipping warm-ups and cool-downs: Getting your body ready for exercise is crucial to preventing injuries and getting the most out of your workout. You put a lot of strain on your tendons, ligaments, joints, and muscles when you strength train.

For this reason, it is essential to start work with a five- to ten-minute warm-up. A few dynamic stretches, such arm circles, leg swings, and hip circles, should come after a five-minute aerobic warm-up, such as walking, high knees, or running. After your workout, allow your body to cool down for five to ten minutes by performing some low-intensity aerobic exercise and static stretches.

Overtraining and inadequate recuperation: In functional strength training, overtraining can lead to injury and burnout. If you engage in intense, ongoing training without taking proper breaks, you may develop overtraining syndrome. The signs of overtraining syndrome include increased resting heart rate, decreased motivation and desire to train, and degradation of physical performance. Diseases and injuries are becoming increasingly frequently. Appetite changes, disturbed sleep, and irritability: To prevent overuse problems and optimize your progress, give your body enough time to rest and recover in between workouts. Erroneous form and technique can cause injuries and reduce the effectiveness of the exercises. It's imperative that you master the correct form for every exercise and maintain it throughout your training sessions. See a professional personal trainer or strength and conditioning coach if you have any questions about how to do certain functional strength training exercises.

There's not enough diversity or advancement. Functional strength training should incorporate progressive overload approaches, such as progressively increasing the resistance, intensity, or complexity of exercises, to keep your muscles challenged and help you continue to make progress. To push your body in different ways and engage different muscle groups, you should also modify the way you move. FAQs Regarding Functional Strength Training: What is the recommended frequency of performing functional strength training? Functional strength training is a great full-body workout since it works all of the major muscles in your body. Compound or multi-joint exercises are a common feature of regimens, allowing for the utilization of larger loads. It is crucial to give yourself time to relax in between sessions as a result. You should take one to three days off in between functional strength training sessions, depending on your current training condition.

Can functional strength training be combined with other forms of exercise? It is possible to mix functional strength training with other types of physical activity. This workout can be used to complement stretching, other forms of exercise like yoga and Pilates, and cardiovascular routines because it consists of compound movements that target the body's primary muscles. How long does it take to see effects from functional strength training? It's hard to say for sure how long functional strength training will take to show improvements. At first, it's normal to feel happier, less stressed, and get higher quality sleep.

Nevertheless, it could take a few weeks to notice and experience gains in strength. What distinguishes traditional strength training from functional strength training? While single-joint and multi-joint exercises are frequently included in workout routines for traditional strength training, multi-joint or compound motions are given priority in functional strength training. Exercises that only use one joint include the triceps extension, seated leg curl, and biceps curl. Although functional and traditional strength training have distinguishing characteristics, you can incorporate both into your entire training regimen.

Bottom Line: If you're searching for a fresh approach to exercise, functional strength training may be the answer. With the help of multi-joint exercises that work several muscle groups at once, you may concentrate on movement patterns that closely resemble everyday tasks and enhance your general strength and mobility.

It's simple to begin functional strength training! Before you hit the gym, just make sure your body is prepared and you have the necessary knowledge. Speak with your doctor, get advice on good form from a trainer, and make sure functional strength training is part of your entire fitness regimen are some things to think about.

Chapter 2

Functional Movements vs. Traditional Exercises

While light cardio is usually a decent place to start when working out at the gym, what should you do next? You might want to think about lifting weights to build strength. Strength training is a great workout, even for beginners. It contributes to the increase of flexibility and mobility, the decrease of stomach fat, and cardiovascular health.

 It also raises your vitality and attitude. So which kind of strength training—conventional or functional—should you prioritize? It could be challenging to distinguish between the two if you're a novice. On the other hand, your choice ought to be guided by your exercise objectives. Let's try to understand the differences between the two kinds of strength training sessions. When you think about strength training, what comes to mind? The majority of individuals consider the following when considering strength training: Weightlifting and bodybuilding: In order to build a big body, this type of workout concentrates on working certain muscles.

You won't always use all of the muscles you exercise to exhaustion in your regular life. Circuit and Machine Training: Large gyms often have a lot of equipment designed to work specific muscles alone, which might help with bodybuilding or physical rehabilitation. If you're not into bodybuilding, they might not be of much use to you. A range of barbell exercises are part of powerlifting, a sport for elite weightlifters who are also highly skilled athletes. Conversely, powerlifting could not help you much in your day-to-day tasks or in your overall athletic performance. Moreover, it is not the best option for beginners or intermediate exercisers who want to improve their general level of fitness. What Separates Functional Strength Training from Conventional Strength Training You're not alone if strength training seems unachievable because it falls under one of the aforementioned categories. While these are instances of traditional strength training, there are other methods for building strength as well.

An other choice is functional strength training. This is a thorough analysis of the two. What does typical strength training entail? Using standard resistance training or weightlifting techniques, traditional strength training aims to build larger, stronger muscles. It involves employing exercise bands, weight machines, and free weights to isolate and train certain muscles. This type of strength training uses heavy weights and equipment to work individual muscles until they are exhausted. Three to five sets of exercises, with eight to twelve repetitions each set, can be included in a standard strength training session. These workouts frequently use simple movements.

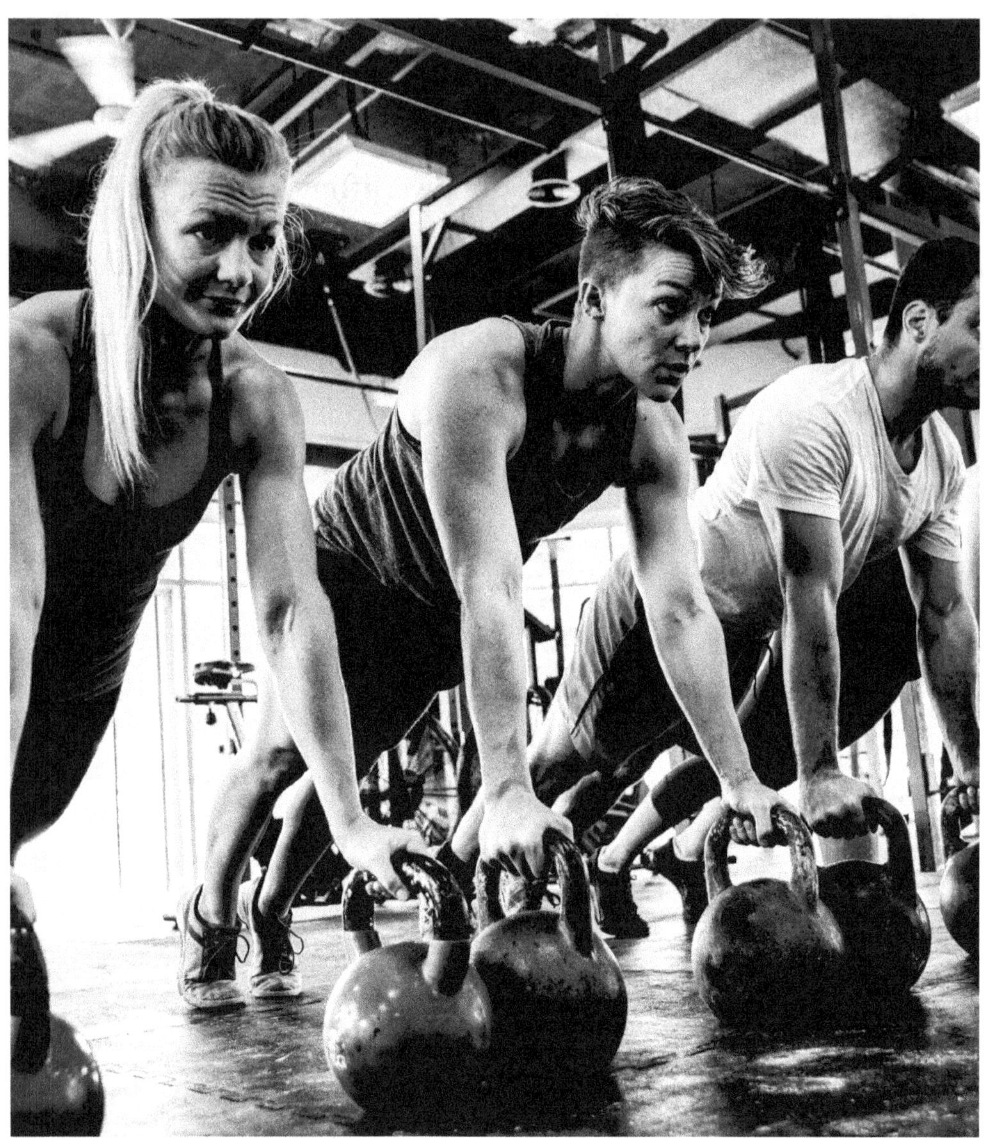

such as curls, rows, or presses that target a particular muscle at a time. Heavy weights are used to test the muscles and create strength. What exactly is functional fitness for strength (FST)? Functional strength training, in contrast to traditional strength training, emphasizes workouts that incorporate daily movements. It improves your body's ability to perform daily activities like going upstairs and bringing groceries into the kitchen. useful training emphasizes full-body workouts that are more dynamic than traditional strength training, even though all forms of strength training are theoretically useful since they improve your physical strength and capacity to perform daily tasks. It strengthens a variety of muscles in one workout, enhancing balance, endurance, and core stability.

For your functional exercise, you can use medicine balls, kettlebells, dumbbells, sandbags, bands, bodyweight, or any combination of these. Planks, push-ups, and side lunges are good basic exercises that work several muscle groups and build strength throughout the body. Increase the difficulty of your workout by adding weights or selecting more challenging exercises like burpees, renegade rows, or rotational lunges.

Common Benefits of Strength Training for Function The following benefits of functional strength training could be obtained by you: Strength and muscle mass growth. The bones are fortified. effectively burns calories and raises metabolic rate to burn fat all day. enhances emotional well-being and mental health It improves your endurance and cardiovascular health. What distinguishes the two from one another? You can improve your mood and your ability to burn fat in addition to gaining more muscle and strength with either type of strength training. Nonetheless, they are differentiated by a few important points. Conventional training involves short sets of focused, accurate movements. In contrast, functional training can be performed in sets, circuits, or HIIT and incorporates many muscle groups into a single exercise. For novices, traditional training is usually a smart alternative because it doesn't need you to stabilize multiple joints at once, which reduces your risk of injury. Conversely, functional training is more widely available because it requires little equipment and can be performed with simple tools like kettlebells and resistance bands. It improves one's ability to do a range of dynamic motions that help with daily work rather than focusing only on one particular muscle group.

What Distinguishes Functional Strength Training Exercises from Conventional Strength Training? Generally speaking, traditional strength training consists of simple yet challenging exercises done with the use of benches, heavyweights, cable pulleys, and sitting machines. More complex training is probably functional strength training. Monitoring your heart rate is also a smart idea when working out. If it increases to more than 70–80% of your maximum, you are undoubtedly engaging in functional strength training, which raises your heart rate and burns more calories. On the other hand, traditional strength training is more likely if your heart rate is lower and you can talk clearly while working out. The growth of muscular and general strength is aided by both traditional and functional strength training. They also help you to improve your mood, increase your body's ability to burn fat and increase metabolism, and support healthy bones. Conversely, functional training consists of exercises that educate the muscles how to work together.

It incorporates everyday motions made while carrying out routine duties. Functional strength is the goal of functional training, which is usually more challenging. On the other hand, traditional strength training concentrates on strengthening certain muscle groups separately. Upon finishing your aerobic workout or treadmill run, you might wish to pick up some weights and engage in strength training. Thus, is it better to engage in functional strength training or traditional strength training? Everything is dependent upon your search parameters. If you want to tone your arms while standing still, the traditional method is recommended. Perform three rounds of bicep curls. Functional training could be your thing if you enjoy performing a series of lunges and squats while holding a kettlebell.

A lot of people combine traditional and functional training methods in their strength training regimens. In fact, the two worlds are blending more than ever, with many gym-goers combining both disciplines to meet all of their fitness goals, according to NASM-certified personal trainer Nolan Parker. Which kind of exercise you choose—conventional or functional—will also depend on how fit you are. According to Lesley Wu, a certified personal trainer at WORKOUT, "most people will start with traditional strength training because it is easy to follow and learn." Wu made this statement to Bustle. He continues, referring to moves like the "farmer's walk," by saying that "functional strength training requires more knowledge and experience to execute specific exercises properly." The following features and benefits of each strength training method will assist you in making your decision. Strength Training the Conventional Method If you want to tone a specific muscle area, like your legs, glutes, or stomach, traditional strength training might be a good option. As stated by NASM-certified personal trainer Natasha Funderburk, "traditional strength training is when you work on building strength or muscle bulk through standard weight lifting or resistance training methods." To isolate one muscle at a time, this involves utilizing exercise bands, free weights, and weight machines. When someone says they're heading to the gym for "leg day," they most likely mean to work out with traditional strength training equipment. That way, "a gym-goer typically breaks up their training week into three to five workouts where a specific area of the body is the emphasis of each workout," says Parker of this methodology.

"This style of training often focuses on muscle hypertrophy, where the user performs three to five sets of eight to 12 reps." The goal is to select a weight that, by the end of your repetitions, will cause your muscles to get fatigued (or stronger). Benefits of Conventional Strength Training Funderburk asserts that traditional strength training is ideal for anyone wishing to gain mass in a particular muscle. "Traditional strength training is also good for athletes and those who are working towards a goal," she stated. For example, adding glute exercises to a runner's regimen can be beneficial. Conventional strength training has also been shown to increase bone density by improving joint mobility and applying positive stress to your bones. All of it, in Funderburk's opinion, contributes to a decreased risk of injury because you're teaching your body how to maintain itself more firmly and physically. Strengthening your functional strength Conversely, functional strength training emphasizes movements that will improve your body's ability to function in everyday circumstances. Everything seems easier when you start a functional strength training program, even carrying groceries and climbing stairs. For illustration, think about groceries.

"Training through functional movements with exercises like the farmer's walk or suitcase carry can come in handy when you want to make the single trip inside with your groceries," Wu stated. "As the name suggests, functional strength training focuses on executing everyday functions with more ease." Long-time exercisers may find functional strength training appealing because these motions are also more dynamic, according to Funderburk. Unlike a "leg day," a functional routine will work multiple body regions, whereas traditional strength training focuses on one isolated exercise at a time. Functional Strength Training's Benefits Strength training programs increase bone density, range of motion, and joint mobility. Functional training, however, might be more useful in day-to-day situations.

According to Wu, functional strength training exercises like farmer's walks, lunges, and squats give your body a strong core, which makes everything appear easier. He notes, "There is unquestionably advantage to both techniques for all types of people: both athletes and non-athletes may gain from strengthening their bodies and practicing more dynamic movements to aid in day-to-day living.

Evaluation and Establishing Objectives

What exactly is a smart goal?

You can also utilize the SMART goal-setting strategy to help you more effectively reach your fitness goals. The acronym for specific, measurable, achievable, relevant, and time-bound is called SMART. Let's examine each SMART element in more detail: Particular For strength training to be successful, it is imperative to have clear goals. Rather than aiming for a broad goal like "becoming stronger," identify the specific area you wish to strengthen. You could aim to accomplish eight pull-ups without assistance or increase your bench press by ten pounds, for instance. You'll be able to comprehend your expectations more clearly as a result. Quantifiable Monitoring your progress is essential to keeping track of your achievements. Instead of just lifting heavier weights, set measurable objectives, such as increasing your squat weight by 20% or lowering your mile run time by one minute. Reachable Be fair and consider your current level of fitness while establishing goals.

We should aim for goals that are difficult but still attainable with consistent effort. After all, you don't want to put yourself in a position where you fail. Applicable Make sure your goals for strength training align with your overall fitness aspirations. Think about your motivations for wanting to get stronger. Make sure your goals are in line with your values, whether you want to improve your functional strength, confidence, or athletic performance.

Temporal-Based Setting a strict deadline for your strength training goals helps to keep you accountable and motivated. Set a deadline for completing your goals rather than an open-ended one.

Consider the scenario where you have four days to complete a push-up with flawless form. This will help you with goal-setting because you'll know exactly when to achieve the desired outcome. 13 SMART Goal Examples for Strength Training These are some excellent SMART goals for your strength training regimen: 1. Increase maximum deadlift "The person will be able to raise their maximum deadlift in less than six months."

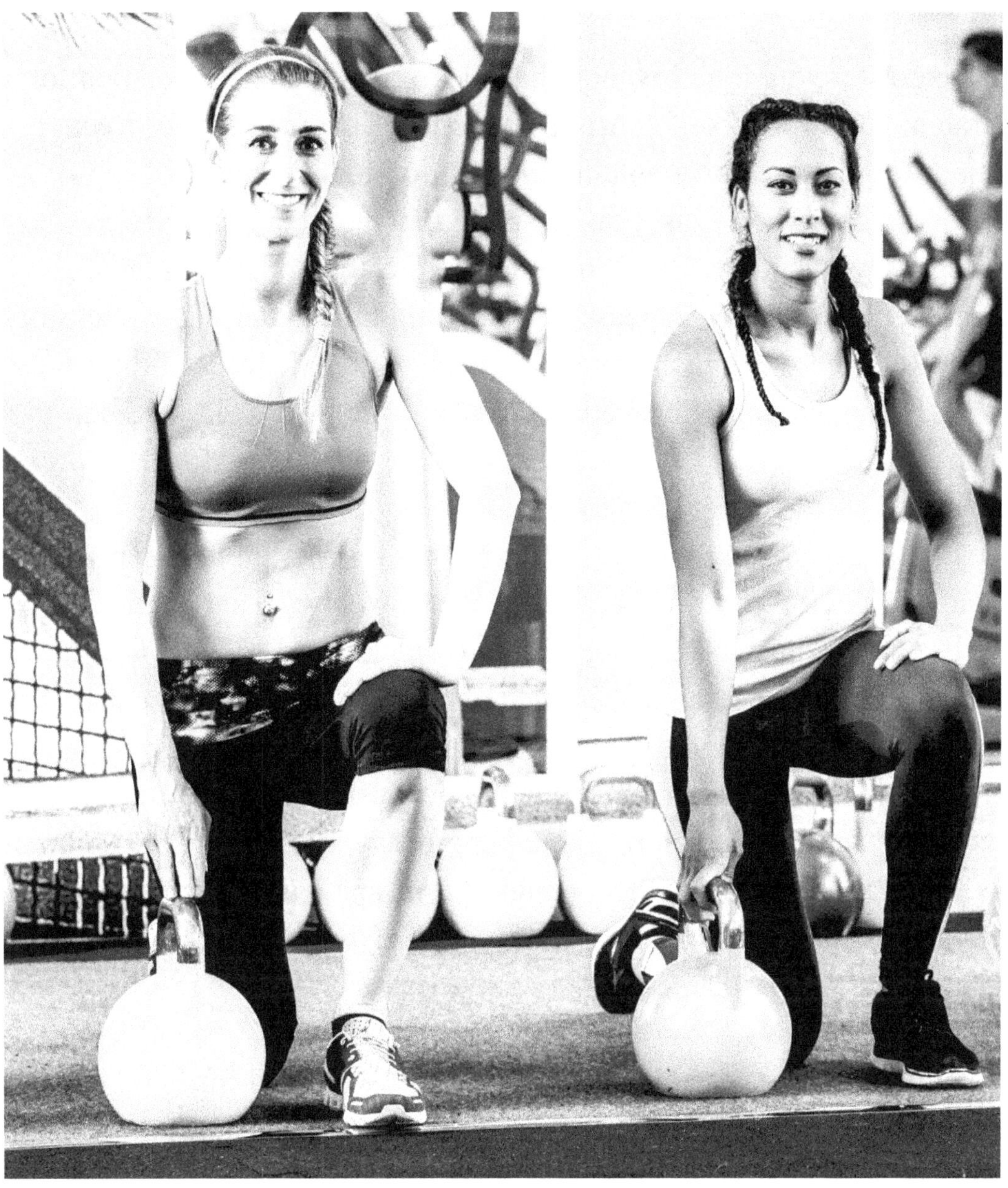

by ten kilograms. "They will train and raise the weight of their deadlifts twice a week."

Specific: The statement outlines your plan to increase your maximum deadlift as well as your goal towards achieving it. Measurable: To monitor your progress, raise the deadlift weight twice a week.

Achievable: Deadlifting is feasible provided you put in the necessary effort and perseverance. Increasing strength and muscle tone requires perfecting the maximal deadlift. Time-based: You have six months to finish the task at hand.

2. Plank holds to bolster your core I want to be able to hold the plank position for 60 seconds straight after 8 weeks of consistent practice. "Three times per week, I will strengthen my core muscles by holding the position for 30 seconds." Particular: The individual knows just how to strengthen their core muscles. Measurable: Regularly record the length of time you are able to hold the plank. Attainable: You should be able to increase your holding times after eight weeks of consistent work. Relevant: Having a strong core helps with balance, stability, and posture when performing tasks. Time-bound: You have the next eight weeks to finish your SMART goal.

3. Shorten Rest Period Between Sets: "I want to cut my rest period between sets from two to one and a half minutes within the next two weeks." That ought to make it easier for me to adjust to working out more quickly and enable me to have more intense muscle-building sessions." Particulars: The objective is to reduce the amount of time rest between sets for the next two weeks. Measurable: This can be evaluated by reducing the two-minute rest interval between sets to one and a half minutes. Attainable: Cutting back on rest hours progressively is within the realm of feasible goals. Relevant: Shortening the amount of time spent at rest increases the intensity of training, which improves muscular growth. Time-bound: There is a two-week deadline for this particular goal.

 4. Find a Strength Training companion: "I'll look for like-minded fitness enthusiasts online and ask around at my local gym within a month to find a strength training partner." "My partner should be devoted to safety, understand appropriate technique, and share my goals." Specific: The goal is laid out with a time frame of one month and the qualities that are desired in a strength training partner. Measurable: One way to measure success is to find a compatible companion. Attainable: It should be easy to locate a suitable strength training partner within the allotted time frame with the right care. Relevant: Getting the most out of each strength training session requires finding a trustworthy and knowledgeable partner. Time-bound: You have to find a training partner after a month.

5. Perfect the one-leg squat "I will master the single-leg squat in three months by attending two weekly leg strength and stability workouts." "I intend to improve my form and gradually increase my weight loads." Particulars: The goal is simple: in three months, master one-leg squats. Measurable: Schedule two leg strength and stability sessions each week. Attainable: This is achievable if the person is patient and follows through on their plan. Relevant: This goal is pertinent to the demands of the individual because single-leg squats are essential for leg strength and stability. Time-bound: Three months are allotted for finishing the SMART statement.

6. Change Up Your Bicep Curls "I want to try three different types of bicep curls to challenge my muscle strength and endurance as I build up my bicep muscles." This will incorporate once-weekly barbell, dumbbell, and hammer curl exercises by the end of four months." Particular: The goal outlines the exercises that will be done and how frequently. Measurable: You might record the quantity and type of bicep curls you perform in a given week. Achievable: Since three curls can be finished in a single weekly session, this is doable. Relevant: This goal is suitable since it emphasizes the development of the biceps and calls for strong muscles. Time-based: Results in terms of fitness take four months to attain.

7. Incorporate plyometric training. "For the next four weeks, I'll incorporate plyometric exercises into my workout routine." I currently work out with weights several times a week, but adding plyometrics to my regimen would make my workouts more intense." Particular: This outlines the kind of exercise that should be incorporated into the fitness routine as well as the completion date of the goal. Measurable: One way to gauge progress might be to keep track of how many plyometric exercises you complete in a given week. Attainable: Since plyometrics are simple to learn and four weeks is a decent amount of time to become familiar with them, this is doable. Plyometric exercises increase general fitness and intensity. Time-bound: It will take four weeks to accomplish this goal.

8. Pay Attention to Various Muscle Groups "I will work on different muscle groups once a week when I do strength training." My current routine emphasizes my back, arms, and chest. For the following twelve weeks, I want to focus on strengthening my legs, shoulders, and core." Particular: The SMART goal outlines the main

objective, the plan of action, and the deadline. Measurable: To target different muscle groups, you can utilize a fitness tracker. Attainable: Since training on different body parts for 12 weeks makes sense, this is doable. Relevant: Since it ensures that you exercise every major muscle group in your body, this is crucial. Time-bound: Within a 12-week period, the objective statement must be accomplished.

9. Carry Out Interval Training "I will employ an online interval training program or sign up for a high-intensity interval training session at the gym to do interval training twice a week for the next two months." Taking an online course or signing up for a class are examples of specific actions. Quantifiable: Ascertain whether you engage in twice-weekly interval training. Achievable: You can raise your level of fitness in two months if you dedicate yourself to the process and work out frequently. Increasing strength and fitness with interval training is highly successful. Temporal: Realistically, you have two months to complete this goal.

10. Firm Your Hold "By the end of three months, I want to increase my grip strength from 70 pounds to 100 pounds by doing finger exercises daily and using a hand gripper twice a week." Particular: This goal lays down what you have to do (finger exercises) and how often you have to do it (daily). Quantifiable: You might compare the amount of weight your grasp can support before and after training. With consistent effort, one can raise their grip strength from 70 to 100 pounds. Gaining more grip strength could make it easier for you to complete exercises like pull-ups and rowing. Time-bound: Within the next three months, goal fulfillment is anticipated.

11. Boost shoulder mobility. "In two months, I'd like to increase my shoulder mobility by 10%." I hope to do this by include shoulder mobility exercises in my daily training routine for at least ten minutes." In two months, a person wants to increase shoulder mobility by ten percent. Measurable: You may track the improvement in your shoulder mobility as you exercise on a regular basis. Attainable: Given that the person has been consistently working to increase mobility for the past two months, this is doable. Relevant: Since the goal will fortify them and help avert shoulder issues, it is appropriate. Time-bound: With a two-month deadline, the goal is time-bound.

12. develop exercises for the upper body. "In the following three months, I will increase my strength in upper body exercises by dedicating at least four days a week to weight training and completing three sets of shoulder presses and lat pulldowns with weights ranging from 10-15 lbs." Particular: The goal outlines the activities that must be performed and the frequency at which they must be completed. Measurable: By raising the workout weight and counting the number of sets performed, one can gauge one's strength. Attainable: This is doable because it outlines a reasonable time limit for reaching the desired outcome. Relevant: Any exercise program must focus on building upper body strength. Three months is the allotted time to complete the SMART goal.

13: Develop Better Pull-Up Form "I want to increase my pull-up max from 10 to 15 by perfecting my form and making sure each repetition is performed correctly." I intend to up the difficulty in the next eight weeks by incorporating a weighted vest into some of my sets." Since the person wants to increase their pull-up maximum, this is expressed clearly. Quantifiable: To gauge your level of fitness improvement, count how many pull-ups you can perform with proper form and if you've completed 15 reps at any given point in time. Realistic: If an individual is consistent and committed to their training, they can complete 15 pull-ups in 8 weeks even with an intermediate level of fitness. Relevant: Since it involves a purpose that will help the person both personally and physically, this is pertinent to them. Time-bound: You have eight weeks to finish this goal. Final Thoughts Throughout this essay, we have discussed how SMART goals can help increase the success of strength training. Now is the moment to step up and reach your greatest potential.

Just remember to regularly monitor your progress. Having actual data lets you see your progress, whether you're measuring your own weight, recording your repetitions, or monitoring your jogging time. Locate a group of people that are as passionate about strength training as you are, or find an accountability partner. When things go tough, they may support, mentor, and motivate you.

Evaluating Functional Fitness

5 Tests to Assess Functional Fitness Touching Your Feelings
You can assess your current level of performance in this area of function by giving yourself this quick and easy test. Is it possible for you to reach your toes while standing straight-legged, or even better, to place your hands on the ground? Should you be unable to achieve this, your risk of suffering a back injury can increase.

 Other muscles might need to compensate for a restricted muscle during a movement until the restricted muscle is repaired. Toe touching while standing is a great way to identify the issue. SIT-STRENGTH SADDLE This is an additional useful and effective way to measure the range of motion (ROM) between your hips and your groin (adductors). Simple instructions for this test include sitting on the ground and spreading your legs into a "V." Ideally, you should be able to achieve this by holding yourself in place without having to lean against a wall or place your hands on the ground to keep your body upright, and by keeping your spine neutral and perpendicular to the ground (as opposed to bending forward). Seeing if you can complete this action without the assistance I just described is one way to assess your development.

A second way to monitor your progress, if you can do this on your own, is to measure the distance between your feet when your legs are stretched into a "V." Simply mark the inches and feet on a piece of tape that is laid out in a straight line on the ground to measure this. To measure the distance, placing one foot on one end of the tape and the other on the other while you adjust to your position. Additionally, keep your back of your legs pressed into the ground and your knees straight while in the saddle-sit posture. Your feet ought to be flexed as well during the exercise.

The rectangle of the globe Don't undervalue the goblet squat as a potent strength training exercise. Actually, I've witnessed this method demoralize a lot of individuals who thought they were strong in the squat. The goblet squat is a great approach to improve a bad squat pattern and evaluate your squatting technique.

You must perform 25 consecutive squats with a kettlebell or dumbbell that is half your body weight in order to pass the goblet squat exam. You're not ready for a barbell back squat if you can't execute it with a dumbbell or kettlebell. The weight acts as a counterbalance to support you at the base of the squat and forces you to engage your core center for improved squat stability because it is front-loaded and rests on your chest and abdomen.

PULL-UP STRONG

One of the hardest strength workouts you can perform is the pull-up. That being said, another fantastic strength exercise that is overused in many gyms worldwide is the pull-up. As with the goblet squat test, the objective of this functional fitness testing is for you to demonstrate strict execution of the exercise. You should grasp the bar with your hands shoulder-width apart in order to perform the pull-up test. You should start with your arms fully extended and your shoulder girdle almost completely relaxed while you dangle from the bar. After raising yourself to the point where your neck meets the bar, assume a full dead-hang position with your arms perfectly straight. The secret to this workout is precise technique. The exercise has the greatest impact when performed with a tight technique. Being able to perform at least six strong pull-ups with proper form is the objective.

Naturally, it would be great if you could score higher, but even if you don't, this exam will give you a starting point from which to retest yourself following a training cycle.

POWERFUL PUSH-UP

To pass the challenging push-up exam, you must be able to perform at least 12 strict form push-ups at a pace of 60 beats per minute while maintaining an upright push-up stance. You should demonstrate stiffness and the ability to maintain perfect alignment of your body from your shoulders to your ankles when performing the tight push-up. Make sure you can perform full-range push-ups in time with the metronome and maintain proper body alignment, and then record your number.

When you are unable to keep up with the metronome or your push-up form is compromised, the test is done. I advise recording this exam if you're taking it alone so you can evaluate how you do and give yourself a more accurate score.

Chapter 3

Setting Personalized Strength Goals

Prior to beginning any weight-training program, you should establish a clear and detailed set of goals related to your own fitness and well-being. You should have both short-term (one week to less than six months) and long-term (six months to a year) goals for your personal fitness. Determine your own fitness goals by considering the reasons behind your desire to improve your general health and level of fitness.

 Additionally, bear in mind any time or physical constraints while setting your personal fitness objectives. It's important to come up with a set of goals that are challenging but yet realistic and reachable. To get a fit and healthy lifestyle, think about creating your personal fitness goals. It's important to keep in mind that your individual weight training goals should be focused on certain metrics pertaining to your weight, measures, strength, and cardiovascular endurance.

The following suggestions can assist you in establishing meaningful and practical short- and long-term goals: Objectives: Short-Term vs. Long-Term For every three short-term goals, most people will set one long-term ambition. The long-term goal should be accomplished with the aid of the short-term goals. Both short- and long-term goals consist of the following:

Short-Term Goals Over the course of a week, complete three sets of twelve sit-ups on four different days. One meal a month, swap out one meal for a salad. I completed one set on each piece of weightlifting equipment at the gym during my first two weeks there. Long-Term Goals You might shed fifty pounds in eight months. Be able to bench press 180 pounds on a straight, flat bar in less than a year. In six months, grow my biceps to a measurement of 14 inches. Better Weight Training Objective Setting: Advice and Strategies Every person needs to have certain goals.

Ensure that your strength training goals are clear and unambiguous, as they could be interpreted incorrectly based on your performance. For example, setting the objective to be able to perform a 180-pound flat-bar bench press is far more impressive than saying, "I want to improve my fitness level." Every goal ought to be measurable so that it is clear when it has been attained. For instance, you should compute your body fat percentage before to beginning a weight training program and then set a body fat percentage target if your goal is to lower it. For instance, you can set a 6-month long-term goal to reduce your starting body fat percentage of 28% to 20%. You might also set a short-term goal of reaching a 23% body fat percentage in three months. You can review your 3-month goal to make sure you are on track to reach your 6-month long-term goal by setting a short-term goal that matches to a long-term target. Establish reasonable weight training goals that aren't overly basic. A false sense of achievement may arise from objectives that are too easy to achieve, while goals that are too difficult to achieve will probably sap your motivation and possibly even cause you to give up.

Establish deadlines for completing your objectives. You force yourself to continue paying close attention and taking responsibility when you set deadlines for each goal. Both short- and long-term goals must to have an end date in mind. Decide on a timeline in which you will complete any given task. Make use of these deadlines to assist you in achieving your long-term goals. By linking short-term targets (milestones) to long-term objectives, you may determine whether your weight training program is producing the desired results in the time frame you have projected. For instance, you may set four short-term objectives of 15 pounds of excess body fat every three months if your long-term aim is to lose 60 pounds of additional body fat in a year. Setting deadlines for each goal instills a sense of urgency and supports sustained focus and motivation. Clearly define and document your goals in a weight-training journal.

When you see checkmarks next to every goal you have accomplished, it may be a great motivational boost. This lets you track your progress toward various objectives. Establish a precise, step-by-step plan for accomplishing every weight training goal you set. It is imperative to provide a comprehensive explanation of your intended approach for achieving even short-term goals. This task is usually easier if you are currently on a particular weight training program because you can just modify your real workouts.

To find out exactly where you stand in terms of strength and physical dimensions, it is advisable to perform a brief introductory activity before starting a weight training program. For instance, you would most likely miss your target if you set a 6-month aim to increase your biceps measurement to 16 inches and then find out that they are only 12 inches when you first measure them. It's a better approach to measure your biceps first, then set short- and long-term goals.

Try a few different approaches to achieve your goals. There are typically dozens or even hundreds of different ways to accomplish the same goal. Adding variety to your weight training regimen is essential because it will push your body to continually adjust to the demands you put on it, which will help you achieve even better results. An Example of a Goal Chart It's a good idea to set out your goals in a step-by-step manner before beginning an exercise program that involves weight training so that you can begin defining your weight training sessions to achieve your goals.

One of the best tools for accomplishing short-term goals is a target chart. Generally speaking, achieving short-term goals leads to the accomplishment of long-term ones. Stated differently, attaining short-term success can lead to long-term success. Below is an example goal list. Make a note of each goal's detail and clarity. One-week Short-Term Goal: In the first week of training, I performed two full-body exercises.

At 5:00 p.m. on Monday and Thursday, I will work out. On both days, I'll follow this weight-training schedule. There are three sets of exercises. Twelve repetitions in a set. Exercises that need to be finished are: Bench press with a straight, flat bar Rows with a dumbbell held in one arm Presses from the military are placed behind the neck. Curls with a barbell that is standing Extension of the triceps Squats squats using dumbbells crinkles around the stomach asymmetrical twists in the abdomen Short-Term Objective (1 Month): At the moment, I can bench press a flat straight bar 12 times with 80 pounds. My short-term goal is to be able to bench press 100 pounds 12 times with a flat straight bar in one month. I will perform the following workout twice a week in order to reach my goal: I will gradually increase the weight and lower the number of repetitions until I can perform the flat straight bar bench press 12 times with 100 pounds after finishing the exercise below for the first week. Exercises that need to be finished are: Bench press with a straight, flat bar There are three sets in all. 8–12 repetitions for each set There are 12 repetitions of 80 pounds in the first set. The second set consists of 10 reps at 85 pounds. Set 3: 90 pounds until it breaks One year from now, the long-term objective is to be able to bench press 180 pounds 12 times with a flat straight bar.

I plan to continue utilizing my short-term flat straight bar bench press in an effort to approach my long-term objective. Every training session will include three sets of 12 repetitions of the following shoulder movements, in addition to the flat straight bar bench press: front lateral dumbbell raises and military presses performed while sitting behind the neck. Setting short- and long-term weight training goals is a fantastic method to keep focus and motivation high, as was previously said. Actually, you'll find that reaching your own weight-training goals gets easier as your weight-training efforts increase. You'll also find that your drive and focus are elevated, in addition to the achievement of your targeted weight training goals becoming more predictable. Lastly, a lot of people who utilize this method to determine and achieve their own weight training goals also prefer to use it for nearly all other aspects and objectives in their lives.

You can use this tactic, for instance, to improve your financial status, your work performance, or even your relationship with your partner, significant other, or kids. One way to obtain a fit, healthy, and mentally well-being lifestyle is to take the time to create a comprehensive and well-considered set of objectives and then implement an action plan to reach those goals.

Exercises for Functional Strength

A type of exercise called functional strength training concentrates on getting the body ready for daily tasks, sports, or specific occupations. Increasing functional movements and general functional fitness is the major goal of functional strength training. What does that mean exactly? Think about the small movements you do every day: climbing and descending stairs, carrying a shopping bag, and hiding on the ground to play hide-and-seek with your kids. These are all functional motions, and depending on your level of functional fitness, your stamina may be limited.

Strength training that is functional as opposed to traditional Functional strength training uses movements like bodyweight squats and other exercises that mimic real-life motions. Although I enjoy a nice devil's press just as much as the next person, we thankfully don't use it frequently! There is some crossover between traditional strength training and functional strength training. Because functional strength training consists of resistance exercises that challenge the body's muscles, it may increase strength.

Given that increased strength and muscular ability facilitate daily chores, traditional strength training may also somewhat enhance functional fitness. The important thing to remember is that strength training targets specific muscle groups. This could entail motions like: The push of the shoulders Curl your biceps. Bent rows across the glutamine bridge hollow-body hold Exercises for functional strength training include the following examples: Push-ups Jumps from a squat sways to the side when strolling, lunges Deadlifts using just one leg You've undoubtedly come across motions from both categories if you've ever performed a strength workout on Peloton. These two training courses overlap one other quite a bit. When these components are combined, you get a well-rounded workout. Functional Strength Training's Benefits The benefits of functional strength training are numerous. To begin with, it enhances one's ability to perform daily tasks more efficiently. It seems senseless to tense up a muscle while carrying a grocery bag. Your muscles may be strengthened and protected by functional strength training. Additional benefits of functional training include the following: Stability and core strength have increased. For nearly everything, your core is necessary. Sports health studies, however, indicate that you run the risk of injury if you don't engage your core vigorously. Planks and other functional workouts educate you how to use your core muscles automatically.

Better stability and posture result from this. enhanced coordination and balance You could think you were born clumsy if you frequently stumble, lose your balance, or walk unevenly. Most likely, all you need to do is practice your balance. Dynamic exercises (like single-leg deadlifts or reverse lunges) allow you to shorten and stretch your muscles in one motion, which helps your muscles contract and relax. Over time, this might help you become more stable in your daily life, activities, and sports. Preventing Injury Joint stability can be improved and muscular imbalances can be corrected with the help of functional strength training. This reduces the risk of injury from sports or daily activities. For example, functional strength training is important for runners and cyclists to stay in the sport as well as improve performance. Your lower body strength will increase with lunges and squats. You may enhance your running gait and maintain proper cycling posture by strengthening your core with planks.

Hip and Glute Stress A lot of functional strength training exercises focus on the hip flexors and glutes. For runners and bikers, this is crucial knowledge in mechanics. Strong hip and glute muscles can provide you the extra push you require, particularly when running or climbing. Adaptability and mobility Dynamic stretching is a big part of functional strength training (think walking lunges and scapular push-ups). By concentrating on mobility, these stretches will increase your range of motion and flexibility. Additionally, they lessen the chance of overuse injuries. Particularly as you age, functional training is a great way to maintain joint mobility and stay active. Enhanced Burning of Calories Functional strength exercises are more dynamic than isolated strength training, which may lead to a higher caloric expenditure. This is because, as you are working against the opponent, you are increasing your heart rate. Additionally, you're working multiple muscles at once, which uses more energy than standard strength training, which just works one muscle.

Time Administration You are aware of your potential for effectiveness in a brief amount of time if you have ever completed a Peloton App Flash 15 or 20 Minute HIIT Cardio. Because functional strength training frequently involves complicated motions that target multiple muscle groups at once, it's a great way to get in a rapid workout. Try these exercises for functional strength training. Many of your strength training sessions will include both traditional strength exercises and functional strength training strategies.

If so, that's great to hear! Functional strength exercises help you develop your endurance in addition to strengthening your muscles through isolation. Here are some exercises to get you started if functional strength training is something you have never done before: First, squats With your knees slightly bent, place your feet hip-width apart. As though you were seated in a chair, slowly lower yourself while activating your core. Verify that your knees are not giving way under you. After three to five seconds of holding, slowly move back to the starting position. Make it harder. From a squat position, extend your legs by engaging your core and driving through your feet to make a leap. Quickly squat again after landing lightly on the balls of your feet. 10 repetitions is the desired amount, which is equal to 5 standard squats and 5 squat jumps. 2. Makes an opposite-directional lunge Place your hands on your hips and place your feet shoulder-width apart to start. With your left foot, take a large stride back while bending your knee as much as you can toward the ground. This will engage your core. There should be a 90-degree angle between your right foot and the ground. Planting your right foot firmly on the ground will bring you back to starting position.

Perform 10–20 alternating reverse lunges on the left and right, 5–10 on each side. 3. Single-leg deadlifts Arrange heavy dumbbells, approximately 15 to 20 pounds, in a horizontal fashion between your feet and maintain a shoulder-width distance between them. Start this workout with just your bodyweight if you've never done it before. Lean forward, putting your left leg out in front of you and shifting your weight onto your right foot. As you drop your arms to the center of your shins, raise your left leg while keeping a slight bend in your right leg. Using your glutes and core, slowly bring yourself back to the starting position. After five to ten repetitions, swap legs. Fourth: Push-ups In a high plank position, place your hands beneath your shoulders and your feet shoulder-width apart. Maintaining your elbows close to your body, slowly lower your chest until it just touches the mat, or as close as possible. Ascend gradually to your starting high plank position, keeping your elbows pointed inward toward the mat instead of outward. With the right form, aim for five to ten repetitions. For beginners, modify this movement by starting at your knees and working your way up. Five reps of burpees Drop your hands to the floor outside of your feet and start in a squat. Jump or take a step back to get back into a push-up or high plank position. Do one push-up. With his feet outside of his hands, the frog leaps. After doing one squat leap, return to your beginning squat position. Aim for five to ten reps without stopping. Step-ups are the sixth Step up with your right foot first and your left leg second, utilizing a box, small chair, or stool. Lower your right foot and bend your right knee first, then your left. After five to ten repetitions, swap legs. Make it more challenging: Hold dumbbells weighing 10 to 15 pounds in each hand as you go. 7. Board Start in tabletop position, with your neck in line with your spine and your shoulders heaped over your wrists.

Tuck your toes and extend your feet behind you to form a full plank position. Maintain a stable posture while using your pelvic floor muscles. Functional Strength Training with Peloton Try including two or three times a week of functional strength training into your workout regimen, regardless of your current level of fitness.

Functional strength training might enhance, not replace, your preference for strength training. While functional strength training enhances the usefulness of that strength in daily motions and tasks, strength training is useful for focusing on specific muscle groups and maximizing strength.

Core Exercises for Stability

Fit experts who think the term "core" is gimmicky would rather use terms like "trunk," "center," or "column." Some find the phrase offensive due of its imprecise meaning.

Here's a straightforward—though somewhat unsettling—way to see the core: "Unplug" the head, legs, and limbs, and you're left with just the core! To be more precise, the lumbo-pelvic-hip complex and other muscles pertaining to the spine are collectively called the "core of the core." The LPHC includes the hip joints, pelvic girdle, abdomen, and lumbar spine. Any muscles that cross over or directly affect the LPHC are considered core muscles (NASM 2018). Whatever you call it or how you see it, fitness professionals need to understand its movements and function because this body part serves as the foundation for almost all other movements. The arms and legs cannot produce the necessary force or speed for an activity if the core is not strong enough to support it. Reducing belly fat and improving stability are vital! Fitness experts claim that this is the reason why every action serves as a core exercise. As we learned in our core training course, let's get into the specifics of core training. A LOGICAL AND PROGRESSIVE METHODS FOR CORE TRAINING Like any good regimen, a core training program needs to be designed so that exercisers progress safely and logically, providing a strong foundation (figuratively speaking) before adding strength or power workouts.

Trainers and clients frequently forego the stabilization phase in favor of more energizing and stimulating movements. Limitations in core stability training can affect structural and movement efficiency, performance outcomes, and ultimately cause pain or injury. In reality, some patients may have back pain due to a lack of core stability and mobility; providing appropriate core strengthening activities can assist to relieve this pain (Gomes-Neto et al. 2017). While we cannot treat or eliminate pain, as personal trainers we can assist with deficiencies in stability and mobility. For example, we will approach a postpartum client differently than when we recommend postpartum core workouts. Evaluations for stability and mobility restrictions are crucial because every customer is different.

Optimum Performance TrainingTM (OPTTM), a paradigm proprietary to NASM, offers a path to enhance functional skills like cardiorespiratory endurance, flexibility, balance, strength, and core stability. We'll examine stability, strength, and power in connection to fundamental training in the OPT paradigm of NASM in this post. Assessing the Strength of a Client It is essential to comprehend how the spine moves in order to comprehend the core. The spine can flex laterally in the frontal plane (side bend), flex and lengthen in the sagittal plane, and simultaneously combine these actions in and across many planes (as in a crunch with rotation). Starting a core training program at the maximum level the client can retain stability while performing an exercise with proper form is a good idea.

The presence or absence of core stability can be ascertained by a variety of movement assessments. These are a few, by no means all-inclusive, options: test of double-leg lowering Evaluation of overhead squats and pushups (OHSA) Quadrupedal opposite arm or leg raise (dog-bird) (spine not rounded or arched) When a client is ready to move on to more vigorous core exercises, reassessments are utilized to review the client's progress and status. Put this video on hold for later if you're still not sure how far you should push core training for your clients. Crucial Elements of Core Stability: GETTING IN and POSING The two main types of core stability are lumbo-pelvic stability and intervertebral stability. The ability to lessen intervertebral movement is known as intervertebral stability.

This can be accomplished with smaller muscles, such as the multifidus, pelvic-floor muscles, diaphragm, and transverse abdominis. Two exercises include Kegels and drawing in, which involves pressing the navel into the spine. Lumbar-pelvic stability refers to the ability to restrict movement between the pelvis and ribs. This could be aided by abdominal bracing, which isometrically tightens the core muscles. Since drawing-in action and abdominal bracing are essential for performing core workouts safely and effectively, start core training by teaching clients these techniques. WORKING CORE STABILIZATION EXERCISES Stabilization is the first phase in core training, as per the NASM OPT paradigm. At this point, there is very little to no spine motion.

Using this fundamental guideline will enable us to provide a taxonomy for exercise more easily. Anti-rotational exercises like the plank (prone iso-abs) might be incorporated. side plank (side-mounted isoabs) As long as the spine is not sinking or becoming hyperextended, a cobra on the floor with no spinal extension anti-rotation cable for the floor bridge Pallof Press: a standing or kneeling chest press While not exclusively focused on the core, some core-integration activities do require a strong and stable core. For instance: Bend-over pushups in rows kettlebells in a swing Unbalanced loads in deadlifts and carries Just because core stability exercises are the first part of a progressive program does not mean that they are easy. They could be very challenging to complete, let alone correctly. It is easy to increase the difficulty of these exercises by using unstable instruments, perturbations, and other force directions.

WORKING CORE STRENGTH EXERCISES Exercises that target core strength encompass a wide range of spinal motion as well as the entire spectrum of muscular action, including concentric, isometric, and eccentric movements. These movements include flexion, extension, lateral flexion, rotation, and a mix of these joint actions. This is when most people start working out and rarely stop. Here are a few instances of common exercises: Side bends and trunk rotations are compressed by back extension. These core-focused exercises can be made more challenging by incorporating free weights, medicine balls, bands, and cables. There may also be twists like back extensions and rotations with medicine balls and cables. "Exercises for core stabilization are not easy, even though they are the first in a progressive program. They might be quite challenging to complete, and even more so to do correctly. Core Power Exercises Exercises focused on building core power use little to no resistance and emphasize the rate of force production (speed) of the exercise. These workouts are popular with trainers and most consumers since they often involve throwing objects!

 The following are a few instances of exercises commonly done with a medicine ball: rotational chest pass overhead crunch throw A medicine ball pounded into a football toss Throw the ball against a sturdy surface (no drywall!) and use the appropriate kind of ball (such as a wall-ball variation of a medicine ball). Even though the explosive concentric phase is emphasized in power training, we cannot accomplish this without eccentrically lengthening, or stretching, our muscles. The idea is to transition from the stretching phase to an explosive concentric action as fast as feasible. With proper core stability and balance, we can support all parts of the muscular action spectrum, establishing a stretch-shortening cycle and high-functioning integrated performance paradigm (NASM 2018).

A Science-Based Exercise Numerous studies "support the role of core training in the prevention and rehabilitation of low back pain," despite concerns expressed by those in and outside of the fitness industry regarding the potential negative effects of core workouts on the lower back (NASM 2018). Thus, there's no reason for you or your clients to be afraid of core exercises. Exercises that cause discomfort in the back should be avoided, including core stability exercises like planking, core strength exercises like crunches, and core power exercises like rotating chest passes. Otherwise, these exercises are appropriate when combined with a logical, progressive, and well-designed training program, like the NASM OPT model. In actuality, those who adhere to this kind of training may develop core muscles that safeguard the spine during workouts and regular tasks. You will probably be asked these questions at some time in your career, so be ready with these answers! Could I work my ABS every day? Like all muscles, the rectus abdominis, erector spinae, obliques, and other core muscles require time to recover from intense training sessions. You will be training your core to some extent in every functional exercise because it is a necessary component of all of them. But if you work out your core more hard and focused one day, take the next day off to allow your core to recover. ARE THE "LOWER" AND "UPPER" ABS REALLY THERE? Just in terms of place; not in terms of purpose. Does an escalator, for instance, have an upper and lower section? Yes, but just like the rectus abdominis, the escalator works as a single unit. As the phrase goes, "feelings aren't facts." People may feel their "lower abs" during leg lifts and knee tucks. That sensation is produced by the psoas muscles, which attach to T12–L5. The rectus abdominis is placed beneath the psoas muscles. WILL I GET A SIX-PACK FROM CORE TRAINING? It is not a good idea to work on core muscles "so I can see my abs." Only somewhat, core muscles do hypertrophy. Additionally, until they remove belly fat, there's little to no chance that customers will notice their abs. Although core exercises can improve performance and function, decreasing weight will make your abs stand out more.

ADVANCED CORE WORKOUT TEMPLATE The following software was built using the NASM OPTTM model: NASM recommends performing core exercises prior to resistance training, following the warm-up, and early in the workout to activate or "wake" the core muscles. But, as this defeats the purpose, core workouts performed before to weight training shouldn't be performed to exhaustion.

 LEVEL 1 CORE STABILIZATION consists of one to three sets of ten to fifteen repetitions, each done slowly. Side Planks, or Side Iso-Abs Intentionally use your leg and core muscles to draw in and lift for five seconds. Keep your head, shoulders, hips, knees, and feet in a straight line. Press Cable Pallof Reversible Chest Press Place the grips at chest height and the resistance attached to the side while standing with your feet hip-to-shoulder width apart. (The posture gets narrower the harder it is.) Tighten your core muscles, contract your glutes, and pull in your navel. Press the grips away from the middle of the chest during the exercise to prevent any movement or rotation of the LPHC.

CORE STRENGTHENING EXERCISES AT LEVEL 2–3

sets of ten to twelve slow-moving repetitions. Turning Cables Hip and spinal rotation are part of this stage. The body stays erect with the chest up. Think of the trunk as the top-loading washing machine's perturbator—it rotates on a single axis without tilting.

Stability of Ball Back Extension Place the ball low on your abdomen and brace your feet on a wall or a stable machine. Keeping the glutes and leg muscles tense, flex the spine over the ball and then extend using the erector spinae. Level 3 Core Power Exercises Do two to three sets of eight to ten repetitions as quickly as you can without losing control. To make each workout as fast as the last, use a small amount of weight. If slowness happens, there is no longer a code to speed up the formation of force. Health Care Chest Pass with Ball Rotation Less weight (a ball) is used in this progression from the cable rotation exercise to enable an explosive throw, which is how power is produced. Place your feet parallel to the wall and stand sideways, three to five feet away from it. Turn your torso 90 degrees so that your chest faces the wall, then forcefully toss the ball against the wall. (Pick a ball that, in the event of a collision, won't damage the wall.) Smashing a ball of medicine This is an excellent core power exercise because the core serves as the link between an intense upper- and lower-body movement, not because the spine is moving a lot. Lift the medicine ball and place it over you. The ball should then be accelerated to the floor or mat using your entire body.

Chapter 4

The Full Body Functional Movements

We comprehend. It is useless to try to rank the "world's best functional exercises". What distinguishes a thruster from a handstand push-up or a jump squat? The rankings don't really matter all that much. Our intention is to give you ten fantastic, significant, and tried-and-true functional motions that you may choose from to improve your movement patterns, body awareness, and overall strength.

Although there may be disagreements regarding the order, including the exercises on this list in your programming will help you get fitter and run faster. The tenth spot is Farmer's Walk. The muscles targeted are the calves, quadriceps, hamstrings, shoulders, and grip strength. This is as easy as it gets: you are testing your ability to move big, awkward objects around for a long time without dropping them. Long-range grip strength like this is helpful for tasks like unloading all of your groceries in one trip or performing vicious pull-up repetitions or chipper-style deadlift workouts. To Take Action: Hold a large dumbbell or kettlebell in each hand and draw your shoulder blades back and down to stabilize your shoulders. Maintain a tight core, a raised chest, and an upward gaze as you move forward with even, steady steps for the duration of the walk. Expert Advice: "When learning the farmer's walk, use quick, short steps," says trainer Teri Jory, who developed the Poise technique and is located in Los Angeles. "As you get comfortable, you can move faster and lengthen your steps, leading with your hips." 9. Climbing Up the Wall Core, traps, triceps, and shoulders While performing a handstand push-up free-standing is amazing, a handstand push-up against a wall works just as well if you lack the gymnastic bend. It works your shoulders and triceps while also engaging your core and upper body stabilizers to help you stay balanced.

To Do: Spread your hands shoulder-width apart on the floor, about a foot away from a wall. Step one foot at a time into a handstand, or ask a partner to help you, and hold this position with your feet together, your body straight, and your heels touching the wall. Bend both elbows slowly and with total control to lower yourself as far as you can without letting your head touch the ground while maintaining a straight forward gaze rather than looking down at the ground. As you take a step back to the beginning position, keep your core tight. "Practice holding a handstand against the wall for 10 to 20 seconds for three to six sets before going for a push-up," advises Carla Sanchez, the owner of Performance Ready Fitness Studio in Lone Tree, Colorado and a former IFBB Fitness pro. Continue practicing this for a few weeks until you can perform push-ups inverted with ease. eighth. Pull-ups Biceps, middle back, upper back, and lats are worked. An exercise that builds strength and functionality is the back-primed pull-up. How to Do It: Take a wide overhand grip on a pull-up bar and hang freely while crossing your ankles behind you and extending your arms fully.

Lift your body forward until your chin crosses over the bar by drawing your shoulder blades together and pushing your elbows down and back. After a brief period of holding, slowly return to the beginning. "The pull-up is tough, but as you get stronger, you can make it even harder by using ankle weights, changing up your form, or adding in knee tucks," says Samantha Clayton, a personal trainer, former Olympic competitor, and vice president of worldwide sports performance and fitness at Herbalife Nutrition. 7. The Maker of Women Targeted muscles include the quads, hamstrings, glutes, lats, upper back, middle back, chest, and shoulders. This move is a tough, rut- (and gut-)busting workout that incorporates many functional exercises (burpee, renegade row, push-up, squat clean, and overhead press).

 How to Do It: Crouch down and place two dumbbells at your sides, parallel to the floor in front of you. Hold onto the dumbbells while you bounce your feet backward into a plank and then perform a push-up. Keep your elbows close to your torso as you perform a one-arm row on each side while holding at the top. Perform another push-up before jumping your feet back beneath you. As you stand, shrug at full extension and flip your elbows under to bring the dumbbells to shoulder level. Pull the dumbbells up along the front of your body.

Lower yourself to a full squat, then explode upward, raising the weights above your head as you stand. Expert Advice: Patricia Friberg, creator of the DVDs Belly Beautiful Workout and Bottom Line & A Core Defined, says, "This exercise requires a good connection to your core and gluteal muscles." "Do some glute activation exercises in your warm-up, such as squats with a resistance loop above the knee, to prepare for this move." Push/Pull Sled Targeted muscles include the lats, middle back, hamstrings, calves, shoulders, triceps, and biceps. Pushing is a normal human activity that works practically every muscle in the body.

 When combined with a loaded sled, this combo gets you going. To Take Action: Fasten a rope to one end of a sled that is loaded. Stand in front of the sled shoulder-width apart and extend the rope along the floor. Holding the rope tightly with your back straight, lean away from the sled while maintaining a firm grip with both hands. Pull the sled toward you, hand over hand, until it reaches your feet. Then, using strong, steady steps with your hands on the uprights, push the sled back to the starting position with your hips low and your elbows bent. Sanchez says, "This is high-intensity training without the high impact." "Load the sled with heavy weight to build strength and power, or use lighter weight and move with more velocity for conditioning benefits." 5. One-Armed Kettlebell Snatch Targeted muscles include the hamstrings, quadriceps, back, shoulders, and traps. Bilateral (two-limbed) workouts can lead to imbalances because the stronger, more dominant arm or leg frequently bears an uneven share of the weight. Kettlebell snatching is a functional, unilateral exercise that can help make up for these deficiencies.

To Do: Approach a kettlebell with your shoulders shoulder-width apart. Hold the handle with one hand while extending the other arm to the side, keeping your chest up and bending your knees and glutes back. Quickly get to your feet, pick up the kettlebell from the ground, and pull it straight up along the front of your body in a single, smooth motion. When the weight reaches your shoulder and you feel almost weightless, punch your arm skyward and let the kettlebell roll gently to the back of your wrist. Lastly, raise your arm straight above your shoulder with your palms facing ahead.

Repeat the process to get the kettlebell back on the floor. Before swapping, complete all of your reps on one side. "It's crucial that your movement fundamentals are strong and you have good shoulder stability before attempting this with a challenging weight," says Power Pilates instructor Patrea Aeschliman, CSCS. "If you can, have a kettlebell-certified trainer help when doing it for the first time." The fourth Crab Reach (Thoracic Bridge) Targeted areas include the back, shoulders, chest, hips, glutes, and core. The crab reach helps relieve the effects of prolonged sitting by strengthening and extending key areas, including your lower back, shoulders, hips, and abdomen.

To Do: Bend your legs and sit on the floor with your hands behind you, pointing backward. Press down with your hands and feet to raise your glutes off the floor, and then raise your hips as high as you can. Reach your left hand forward toward the floor while turning your head to look at your right hand. After a little break, start over from the beginning. Keep switching sides. "When pressing up, start with your palms far enough away from your feet to avoid over-flexing your wrist," advises Missy Reder, a yoga instructor, personal trainer, and creator of the AB-EZE core training tool. "Plus, the added space will allow you to get your hips even higher." 3. Leap Forth Target muscles include the quadriceps, hamstrings, glutes, calves, and shoulders. This simple bodyweight exercise teaches your lower body's fast-twitch muscle fibers to fire as they launch you into the air and contract to decelerate you on the way back. It combines the best resistance exercise of all time (squats) with a plyometric component. To Perform: With your arms swung in front of you, stand with your shoulders shoulder-width apart. Quickly descend into a squat by thrusting your hips back and bending your knees to activate your posterior chain. To create height, extend your hips and knees, leap into the air, and reach back with your arms.

Immediately after landing softly, move into the next squat. "Always land with your knees slightly bent and aligned with your hips and ankles," Sanchez advises. "If you add weight in the form of dumbbells, a weighted vest, or a barbell, use no more than 10 percent of your maximum regular back-squat load." 2. Costumes in Turkish Targeted muscles include the quads, hamstrings, glutes, lats, middle back, traps, shoulders, chest, and core. Using all of your major muscle groups, this multi-part exercise moves you from a laying to a standing position while gripping a kettlebell perpendicular to the floor. To Take Action: Lying faceup with your legs extended, hold a kettlebell straight up over your left shoulder with your elbow locked. With your right arm out to the side, look up at the weight. Using your left foot and right hand as support, bend your left knee and place your foot on the floor close to your glutes. Then, roll toward your right side.

As you rise into a half-kneeling position, bridge your hips and bring your right knee beneath you. The next step is to get up. Reverse the steps until you are flat on the floor to return to your starting position. Keep switching sides. Trainer and Dancinerate developer Ilyse Baker of Los Angeles says, "Take your time and keep your eyes on the weight throughout the entire movement." "Concentrate on each segment of the exercise without rushing, and you'll master it much more quickly." 1. A dumbbell thruster Targeted muscles include the quadriceps, glutes, hamstrings, shoulders, triceps, and core. The thruster works your entire body, from your delts to your legs, as you move from a squat to an overhead press, cooperating and lifting weight in a dynamic manner. Regardless of the kind of equipment you choose to use—barbells, dumbbells, kettlebells—a thruster will quickly increase your heart rate. To Take Action: Place your feet shoulder-width apart and hold a set of dumbbells at your shoulders with your hands facing neutrally. Keep your weight in your heels as you firmly push upward after bending your knees and lowering your hips into a deep squat, if at all feasible. Use your upward momentum to raise the dumbbells above your head while you stand.

Lower the weights to your shoulders and repeat. Owner of the upscale Pilates studio Relevé in Ripon, California, Jennie Gall, a trainer, says that this exercise must be performed in a single, flowing motion. "It's also common to hold your breath, but it's necessary for power in this exercise." Squatting, take a breath, then release it at the top."

Using Resistance Bands and Free Weights

Why It Could Be Harder To Resist Using Resistance Bands Or Free Weights To Build Muscle And Boost Cardiovascular Performance... Flexibility? Is latex being pumped? Pumping rubber? Elastic bands don't seem to be as "tough" or catchy as "pumping iron," but that doesn't mean they should be viewed that way. In this part, we'll "weigh in" on the real distinctions and overlaps between resistance bands and free weights. Every type of exercise has a unique set of benefits that are extremely alluring for the development of muscles and more! Key Distinctions Between Resistance Bands and Free Weights: At first glance, there may not appear to be any similarities between an elastic band and a heavy iron dumbbell. But it's surprising to learn that resistance bands and free weights have more in common. Techniques for Resistance Training Let's start with the obvious comparison: resistance bands and free weights are both tools used in resistance training. Resistance training is any form of exercise that increases muscle mass and strength. A fitness regimen should incorporate both strength and cardio exercises because they are both good for your health. Conversely, strength training is the best way to increase lean muscle mass, strength, and metabolic rate. Variables for Progressive Overload/Resistance Progressive overload, which is crucial for building strength and muscular development, is simply the practice of gradually increasing a stimulus during a workout.

Similar to progressive overload, progressive resistance is a strategy for improving muscle force production, or just raising resistance as strength increases. You can modify progressive overload elements including rest periods, load, repetition, and volume with resistance bands and free weights. You may be challenged throughout your whole range of motion using free weights and resistance bands, unlike weight machines that just allow you to perform one movement. Another progressive overload/resistance variable for muscle development is time under tension (TUT). TUT permits you to slow down the repetition of the exercise by using free weight and/or resistance bands.

Muscle Development, Activation, and Strengthening Alright, let's face the big one: using resistance bands for exercise can, in fact, activate, build, and strengthen muscle! It is not surprising that bands have the ability to grow and strengthen muscle given their commonality as a resistance training tool that can apply resistance changes or gradual overload. But don't believe us when we say this... A 2016 meta-analysis that was published in Clinical Biomechanics 2 states that elastic resistance and isoinertial resistance both stimulate muscles in a comparable way. Continuous inertia is a feature of isoinertial exercises, which are frequently performed as flywheel training. This allows for eccentric loading and resistance variation throughout the movement. Elastic resistance bands (ERB) were found to be a useful training tool in a 2017 study that compared multi-joint workouts with conventional resistance-training equipment (CRE). Researchers think that when the bands stretch at the motions' terminal ranges, the differences between ERB and CRE may be significantly lessened, even as quad activation decreases with band usage. Elastic band training may offer equivalent strength increases to typical resistance training across a range of demographics, including the elderly and those with fibromyalgia and osteoarthritis, according to a more recent 2019 meta-analysis published in SAGE Open Medicine5. There are numerous varieties available. Free weights and resistance bands come in a variety of forms to suit nearly any training philosophy. Dumbbells, medicine balls, kettlebells, barbells, and sandbags are a few free weights that are available in different weight ranges. There are also many different fitness varieties of resistance bands available, including glute and recovery bands, tube resistance bands with grips, flat resistance bands, and (small) loop bands. Let's get trivial! Resistance bands vary in weight (and color) based on how much resistance they create when tugged, usually ranging from "extra light" to "extra heavy." To what extent can a resistance band produce resistance? Resistance bands and free weights are both incredibly portable, though one is obviously more so than the other (more on that later). (You'll have to keep reading for the astounding reaction). Unlike mounted equipment, free weights can be moved anywhere you have room for them—from their weight rack to the gym floor. Key Distinctions Between Resistance Bands and Free Weights: Although they may not seem to be similar, resistance bands and free weights do have several notable (and not-so-notable) differences. Dimensions and Weight: Resistance bands and free weights can be easily distinguished from one another based on their respective sizes and weights. Free weights are generally big and heavy (which is their main use), especially steel barbells, dumbbells, and kettlebells. Conversely, resistance bands are thin and light. A complete set of resistance bands could weigh less than the lightest dumbbell on the market and fit into a tiny bag. Trivia time is here! How much resistance, then, is produced by a resistance band? However, Rogue's silver Monster Band is resistant to 200 pounds of force! Cost: To assist you start and expand your dream home gym, there are free weights and inexpensive dumbbells available.

Contrarily, resistance bands are far less expensive and offer greater value for your money in terms of fitness. With a total resistance of 100 pounds, some of the best resistance bands available cost about $20. Weight is the primary determinant of free weight costs; for example, a set of 50-pound dumbbells will cost more than a pair of 10-pound dumbbells.

All things considered, investing in a full weight rack will cost more money than just utilizing resistance bands. A home gym floor is something we recommend building in case you drop a free weight, so keep that in mind as well. Muscle Loading and Resistance Resistance is produced in several ways by free weights and resistance bands. This affects your positioning in order to load the muscle as efficiently as possible. Free weights only provide resistance in one direction, down, since they constantly load muscle by defying gravity. A 20-pound dumbbell will always weigh 20 pounds since the weight load of free weights is constant, hence changing the weight size is required to increase or decrease the weight. Resistance bands load the muscle with increasing resistance the harder you pull by using elastic force to generate varying resistance. Resistance band load is frequently influenced by the band's thickness and degree of stretching. To visualize the formation and transfer of resistance, think about the chest press action. When using free weights, you elevate the weight against gravity's pull while lying on a bench press.

Physics makes it very difficult to target the chest muscles by chest pressing a free weight while standing. You may effectively press a resistance band and target your chest muscles while standing by attaching the band. You can use the handles or loops to push forward while encircling a band around your back. (For more details, go to our instruction on using resistance bands properly.) Functionality: Resistance bands and free weights have different uses, despite the fact that they are both beneficial. In functional fitness training, free weights are frequently utilized to provide resistance and boost total strength. Exercises using only your body weight, such push-ups and pull-ups, incorporate functional stability and balance. Conversely, because they can aid in pull-ups and other progressions, resistance bands may support and enhance functional training in a different way. Because resistance bands are gentler on the joints and ideal for warm-ups and injury recovery, they can also be utilized as prehab and rehab tools. The Benefits of Free Weights Whether you're deadlifting a barbell, throwing a sandbag over your shoulders, or pressing dumbbells with your chest, free weights are some of the most popular strength training equipment. Let's examine what makes using free weights so common. Tracking Objectives: Increasing their lifting capacity is the common aim of weightlifters. Unlike most resistance bands, free weights plainly display the weight of the lifter, allowing them to know how much weight they are lifting.

It is simple to track increasing overload objectively with a precisely defined weight quantity. For instance, it is easier to understand and less confusing to track a marked free weight over a resistance band labeled "heavy" if the goal is to increase one's overhead press strength by twenty pounds. Durable The saying "you get what you pay for" usually holds true when assessing the cost and robustness of the majority of free weights. Although premium dumbbells, kettlebells, and other free weights will undoubtedly cost you more money, they are fairly durable and long-lasting—as long as they are taken care of, that is. Balance and Stability Training: When performing functional fitness training, one can use free weights or their own body weight as resistance. The mobility of each movement attracts different muscles for stability, as opposed to being restricted to the movement path of a mounted machine.

Developing and using stabilizer muscles actively leads to an organic improvement in general balance and core strength. A comprehensive training program must include stability and balance since these skills lead to higher lifts and better daily mobility. Optimal for Strength and Lifting Workouts: Bands are an excellent tool for strength training, but they are not suitable for the six common free-weight movement patterns: push-pull, squat, hinge, lunge, and carry.

Yes, you can carry a resistance band and arrange your body to perform a banded lunge. But by neglecting the actual resistance that gravity applies to a free weight, you are also denying yourself the full benefits of these focused actions. The Benefits of Resistance Bands: Despite their little (but powerful!) size, resistance bands have hopefully already demonstrated their capacities. Of course, our goal isn't to dissuade you from using free weights; rather, it's to lessen any resistance you could encounter when doing out with bands. Free weights are far more expensive than inexpensive resistance bands. They are especially good for beginners who want to give it a try or for those searching for affordable yet efficient exercise options because of their low cost. Portable and Convenient: If you are a member of a gym, you may typically find free weights and resistance bands readily available for use. You may get each of these equipment online or in-store if you want to expand or improve your home gym. But, because of their tiny size and thin shape, resistance bands are the most convenient to transport and store when compared to free weights. Resistance bands are excellent for portable workout and storage. Is using it safe? Every workout carries some risk of injury, especially if you're not warmed up and performing the exercise correctly. Resistance bands are a great way to warm up without making that common fitness mistake. All things considered, you would think that applying a 50-pound weight to your foot would be more uncomfortable and dangerous than applying a resistance band that weighs less than a pound. Additionally, you have more control over your safety than if you tried to press dumbbells heavier than you are physically capable of, which might significantly raise your risk of injury. This is because you control the resistance that the band creates. Versatile: Resistance bands, combined with a single, small band set, may offer the most exercise variety compared to free weights. Additionally, although while resistance bands aren't typically the main focus of a strength-training program, when combined with increasing resistance, they can nonetheless produce comparable muscular activation and development. Because resistance bands increase power, they are frequently used in addition to muscle training to enhance athletic performance.

(Free weights like slam balls can also provide these endurance benefits.) Bands are helpful for mobility training while you focus on achieving deeper stretches. Individualized resistance band and free-weight exercises are used in physical therapy clinics. However, bands might be the best option for home-based programs due to their simplicity and inexpensive cost. Additionally, bands are kinder to joints and less taxing on them, which makes them a safer option for exercise for older adults and those recuperating from injuries. Additionally, studies that have been published in the Journal of Sports Science and Medicine7 indicate that functional training programs, which incorporate the usage of resistance bands, may improve older adults' cognitive function and level of fitness. When Is It Better to Use Resistance Bands vs. Free Weights? Thus, when ought one to utilize resistance bands in place of free weights and vice versa? The fitness levels, goals, and needs of the exercisers mostly dictate the response. Resistance Bands for Novices: We're torn on this one because both resistance bands and free weights offer clear advantages for those who are just beginning their fitness journey. On the other hand, beginners might benefit most from using resistance bands. Before we wrap up, we can't help but believe that the greatest choice for beginners learning how to track their progress in a workout regimen is definitely marked free weights.

It can be challenging to track using rate of perceived exertion (RPE), particularly when starting out with weight training. Conversely, approaching resistance bands is less intimidating than approaching a group of experienced lifters and grabbing a dumbbell—especially if you're unsure of the recommended weight. Additionally, resistance bands are less expensive if you want to give working out at home a try. The type of "best" isn't nearly as important for beginners as developing proper form. The first thing to focus on while starting a fitness journey is good technique, and working with a personal trainer can be quite beneficial. Traveling with Resistance Bands: Have you ever tried to load and move a hundred pounds of dumbbells? Moving from one garage gym to another is not an option, so the obvious solution is to use resistance bands when traveling. Resistance bands are great for workouts in hotels and on the road. With just a band or two, you can get full-body training practically anyplace due to the variety of resistance levels you may generate. Adjustable dumbbells, or resistance bands, are some of the best small exercise equipment items available.

Resistance bands, however, can be the best option if you want variety without having to shell out extra cash for weight benches or other gym equipment. Resistance bands offer a great deal of flexibility, especially when used in conjunction with an anchor point—which may be as simple as a door. Simply stash your completed office or home workout in a drawer, bag, or other secret hiding place. Cardio: Any exercise that involves using a free weight or resistance band can be made more intense by increasing the speed. However, bands may have the cardiac edge due to the resistance diversity and general safety of explosive banded activities. (Using larger dumbbells for squat leaps increases the potential of injury if the weight strays from the lifter's grasp.) Alternatively, using lower free weights for high-volume sets of 15 repetitions or more is a great way to fire all of your muscles and cause a burn in your lungs. For weight training and pure strength, free weights are perfect. Free weights are a clear choice if your main goals are to strengthen your body and do weight training. It is possible to replicate heavy-weight exercises with resistance bands; nevertheless, there is a limit to how much you can deadlift. To get the most out of your difficult workouts, we recommend using a barbell and sufficient weight plates, even though dumbbells and kettlebells may help you gain strength. Although they are helpful for supplementary exercises, resistance bands shouldn't be the main focus of a strength-training regimen.

The best benefits for fitness go to both! Why not have the best of both worlds and avoid having to choose between the two? Exercises with resistance bands include mobility, warm-ups, accessory work, and more. If you're not like resistance bands, then by all means use free weights when the occasion arises. The two can also be combined for a variety of other exercises, such as deadlifts, shoulder presses, bicep curls, and squats. As you work through the workout, you'll feel the effect of the combined weight and steady strain from the resistance band and free weight. Overall, the biggest gains in strength and fitness will probably come from switching between free weights and elastic bands. Ultimately, though, the most important thing is to focus on form and practice consistently, regardless of the equipment you utilize. Conclusion: Resistance Bands vs. Free Weights Both resistance bands and free weights are excellent tools for strength training, despite their obvious size differences. Everybody has the option to experience increasing overload, resistance changes, a full range of motion, and load variations. Your goals and way of life will largely dictate whether you use resistance bands or free weights; experienced lifters seeking to gain strength should go for free weights. Resistance bands, on the other hand, are suitable for travel and small spaces.

Nor do you need to make a decision. In a well-rounded exercise regimen, resistance bands and free weights can be used separately or in combination. Use "pump elastic" or "pump iron" constantly in your training; that's when the fitness benefits become very alluring! What's the difference between resistance bands and free weights? What Advantages Do Weights Offer Over Resistance Bands? Since weights can be objectively identified by their weight quantity, they allow for more objective monitoring. Lifters, particularly those who use free weights, may enhance their physical strength while also improving their stability and balance. Can weights be replaced with resistance bands? Weights can be substituted with resistance bands and other resistance training tools. But a number of factors decide whether or not you should replace them. For starters, we do not recommend giving up your barbell or other free weights if your goal is simply to get better at strength-based activities. On the other hand, if you want to maintain your fitness level while traveling, resistance bands are the "weight" to use. What Is the Band Equivalent in Weight? The sort and thickness of a band mostly affect its weight. For instance, the resistance of Rogue's Monster Bands ranges from 15 to 200 pounds. Rogue, in contrast, has tube resistance bands that range from "very light" to "super heavy."

Preparing Functional Strength Workouts

Acknowledging Functional Fitness Training: Uncovering 12 Functional Fitness Activities to Fortify

The emphasis on practical movement patterns and overall physical benefits of functional fitness training has contributed to its increasing popularity. What's not to love about functional training, which mimics daily tasks to help you focus on increasing strength, flexibility, balance, and coordination? Functional fitness programs focus on improving mobility and stability while targeting muscles that are frequently ignored or underutilized, in contrast to traditional weightlifting regimes that isolate certain muscle groups. This post will cover twelve distinct types of functional fitness exercises to get you started, various functional routines to attempt, and why it makes sense to include functional strength training in your fitness plan. TESTING DIFFERENT FORMATS OF FUNCTIONAL EXERCISES Allow me to classify functional workouts before we delve into specific functional fitness routines.

Bodyweight Workouts: You may modify these workouts to suit different levels of fitness and they just require your body weight. They increase functional strength and endurance by effectively using multiple muscle groups at once. Make use of functional training tools including kettlebells, medicine balls, stability balls, suspension trainers, and resistance bands. By enabling you to focus on specific muscle groups and improving stability, coordination, and functional movement patterns, these devices add some spice to your workouts. Create circuit-style training programs that incorporate agility, cardio, and strength training. By performing a series of exercises with little rest in between, circuit training produces a well-rounded functional workout that improves muscular strength, cardiovascular fitness, and functional ability.

HIIT: High-intensity interval training: Don't let the word "intense" scare you off! Short bursts of intense exertion are interspersed with short rest intervals during HIIT workouts. HIIT programs that include functional activities improve sprinting, leaping, and quick change of direction abilities while also building muscle and endurance. Functional activities rarely need the use of gym equipment, despite the possibility of doing so. Hand weights may be used in functional fitness exercises, for example, but you can benefit from functional training without having access to a treadmill or elliptical equipment.

Four justifications for training in functional strength

If you're still unsure whether you should try functional strength programs, take into consideration these other ways that functional fitness adds value to everyday life.

Actual Examples: Training in functional fitness gets you ready for day-to-day obstacles. Functional strength training increases your capacity to lift, haul, and reach in daily tasks, which enhances your overall functional capacity and quality of life. Enhanced Functional Performance: Training in functional fitness enhances your capacity to do specific movements and tasks with ease and speed.

Whether climbing stairs or playing sports, functional strength training improves performance by boosting strength, power, and coordination. Rehabilitation from Injuries: To aid in the healing process, functional fitness regimens may be developed. Following an injury or surgery, they help in the recovery of movement patterns, the strengthening of weak muscles, and the enhancement of overall functional ability. Don't forget to consult your healthcare provider for individualized guidance and recommendations while recovering from an injury. improved posture and core strength: Increased core strength and stability are the outcome of functional workouts, which significantly engage the core muscles. By promoting excellent posture, supporting improved balance and spinal alignment, and supporting good posture, functional strength training benefits overall postural health and body mechanics.

Try out these 12 different kinds of functional training workouts. While designing a functional training program, balance activities that emphasize the arms, legs, and core. You'll have no trouble creating a functional fitness routine that works for you because each of the twelve exercises in our collection offers a few modifications. For optimal training results, concentrate on maintaining flawless form and moving at a leisurely pace. exercises where the leg squat is the primary focus. To start, place your feet shoulder-width apart and point your toes forward. bending at the hips and knees, keeping your weight in your heels, keeping your back straight, and using your core muscles. Lower yourself until your thighs are parallel to the floor, then push back up through your heels to revert to the starting position. Retain the appropriate alignment of your knees to your toes and refrain from bending your knees inward. With practice, you can add weight with a barbell or hand weights. Squats improve balance and stability and strengthen the muscles in your legs, glutes, and core. Plunges.

Lunges are a great way to improve your balance and lower body strength. Place your hands on your hips and stand with your feet hip-width apart to execute them. Leaning forward with one foot, transfer your center of gravity forward toward your front foot, and bend both knees to create a ninety-degree angle. Push through your front heel to stand back up, then switch to the other side. Add a hop at the top of the lunge exercise or carry weights in each hand to make it more challenging. deadlifting. Deadlifts are a great way to strengthen your entire body and focus on your lower body muscles. Position yourself with your feet shoulder-width apart and hold dumbbells in front of you. With dumbbells, stoop down and adopt an overhand grip. After raising the weights, lower them to the floor.

Make several repetitions of this movement, focusing on your hamstrings and glutes. To increase the intensity, add weight or perform single-leg deadlifts. Advancements. Find a stable, elevated surface that is at least knee height or somewhat higher, like a bench or step. Spread your feet shoulder-width apart and plant one foot in front of the platform. Firmly plant your right foot on the platform and raise your body onto it by applying pressure with your heel. Stretch your right knee and hip while raising your left foot into the air, or raise your left knee for more challenge. After a brief pause, slowly return to the floor while maintaining your balance and control. Repeat the exercise ten to fifteen times, then swap legs. By utilizing hand weights or dumbbells for a weighted step-up, you can increase the difficulty level.

Activities Centering on the Core Planks Planks and side planks are great workouts to strengthen and stabilize your core. With your hands shoulder-width apart and your arms straight, start with a push-up. To increase the difficulty of the workout, try a side plank. Throughout the exercise, remember to breathe correctly and keep your hips from sagging or rising too high. With regular training, planks and side planks can help with back pain relief, posture correction, and the development of core muscular endurance and overall strength. crunches. A simple abdominal exercise that tones and strengthens the abs is the crunch. For the ideal crunch, lie on your back with your knees bent and your feet flat on the floor. Don't tug on your neck as you place your hands behind your head. As you take a breath, lift your head, neck, and shoulders off the floor by using your core muscles. Continue doing this for several times, pausing when necessary.

Try variations like bicycle or reverse crunches for a harder workout. Daily crunches can assist improve overall physical performance and core strength as part of your fitness regimen. spans across the glute. Glute bridges are a great way to work on and strengthen your legs, glutes, and core. Lie on your back with your knees bent and your feet flat on the floor, hip-width apart, to start. To activate your core, bring your belly button in close to your spine. Your body should form a straight line from your knees to your shoulders as you raise your hips off the floor and apply pressure with your heels. As you complete the exercise, slowly return your hips to the starting position while keeping your core controlled. Repeat, increasing the number of reps as you build strength; start with 10–15 repetitions. ACTIVITIES CENTERED ON THE ARM Dips

in the biceps. One exercise that can be done anyplace there is a sturdy surface is the dip of the triceps. Start by sitting on the edge of a bench or chair with your hands shoulder-width apart. Slide your hips off the edge and flex your elbows to lower yourself. By utilizing your triceps to elevate your body weight, push yourself back up to the starting position. Aim for three sets of 10–12 repetitions while performing a few reps. The biceps are curled. A classic exercise to build arm strength and definition is the bicep curl. To perform this exercise, stand with your feet shoulder-width apart and a dumbbell in each hand. Squeeze your biceps at the top of the movement as you raise the weights steadily to your shoulders while holding onto them tightly. Aim for three sets of ten to twelve repetitions by lowering the weights to the beginning position and repeating for a few more reps.

As your strength increases over time, switch up your curls or use a bigger weight for an added challenge. Shrugs off. Shrugs are a great approach to enhance posture and build strength in the upper trapezius muscles. Place both hands on a dumbbell and place your feet shoulder-width apart. Take a moment to raise your shoulders to your ears, then slowly lower them back down. Try to complete three sets of ten to twelve reps each. For added challenge, try utilizing a heavier weight or holding the shrug at the top for a short while before lowering it again. uses an overhead press to press. Presses overhead are a great way to strengthen your upper body and improve your posture. Start by placing a barbell or dumbbell at shoulder height in front of you and placing your feet shoulder-width apart. Lift the weight above your head with your core engaged, then progressively lower it back to shoulder level. As you progress, progressively increase the weight and aim for three sets of eight to ten repetitions. The Carry of the Farmer You must perform an exercise called the Farmer's Carry while standing with your feet hip-width apart and a heavy object in each hand. It works wonders for strengthening grips, enhancing posture, and boosting stability in the body. You may progressively boost the weight to continue challenging yourself. Functional fitness training gives a more holistic approach to strength training by addressing mobility, stability, flexibility, and sometimes ignored muscle groups. Functional fitness training boosts total functional capacity, everyday activities, sports performance, and injury risk by including workouts that imitate real-life motions. Whether you're an athlete, a fitness enthusiast, or just looking to better your daily functioning, adding functional strength training into your fitness program may help your fitness journey and improve your quality of life.

Chapter 5

Strategies for Periodization and Progressive Overload

Muscle growth is one of the many reasons people hire personal trainers. For some people, building physical strength is especially important. Others are more focused on building muscle mass or stamina. Training for progressive overload is required for each of these goals. Find out more about progressive overload, its importance for building muscle, and how to implement it into the workout plans of your clients. Progressive Overload: What Is It? The technique of gradually increasing the strain a muscle experiences during exercise in order to compel it to adapt is known as progressive overload. Growth results from muscle adaptations. This idea is known as the overload principle because it is so essential to building strength through resistance exercise. There are numerous ways to overload the muscles when lifting weights.

Firstly, try lifting a bigger weight. With this strategy, the muscle has to work harder to complete the exercise even with the same number of sets and repetitions. Increasing repetitions while maintaining the same weight is an additional option. You can raise the rep range to 12 to 15 if the typical repeat count is 8 to 10. Studies show that this progressive overload approach encourages muscle growth in the same manner as higher loads.

You can raise reps and sets at the same time. As a result, there is more training. Increasing the duration of the training session or the frequency of the exercise might also result in an increased load on the muscle fiber. Instead of 15 minutes, you may train each muscle group for 20 minutes in the first scenario. In the latter scenario, weight training could be done three times a week instead of twice. Lastly, increasing the duration of the workout raises its intensity. Less time has passed for the muscles to recover before doing a new set or activity. Strengthening results from this.

Additionally, it helps reduce fat if the change between exercises is swift enough. This is the fundamental idea behind progressive overload: enhancing a training regimen in this way. To achieve continued progress over time, it involves making adjustments to certain aspects of the strength training program. The Benefits of Training for Progressive Overload Progressive loading has two main benefits: it promotes muscular hypertrophy and increases the growth of lean muscle mass. This enables your client to continue reaping the rewards of their training.

Indeed, reaching a plateau while training is common. Progressive overload could assist clients who are stopped for a long time in moving forward again. Making progress is necessary to keep motivation high. There isn't much reason to keep up their exercise regimen if they aren't seeing results week after week. This increases the possibility that they will completely give up their regimen. Still, the progress they are making by keeping the muscle under stress inspires them to keep going. They are inspired to continue exercising because they can observe the benefits.

52 overweight or obese female teenagers took part in one of two fitness programs utilizing progressive overload training techniques in a 2019 study. Both groups' participants enjoyed a number of benefits, some of which were listed below: enhanced aerobic and anaerobic capacity enhanced balance and coordination increased strength in the ankle dorsiflexor, plantar flexor, and knee extensor enhanced functional strength in the lower extremities enhanced manual dexterity Progressive overload may also help older, pre-frail females, according to a 2020 research published in The Journal of Frailty and Aging. This is especially true after

the connection between training and functional motions is established. For example, squats may facilitate sitting on and rising from the toilet.

Progressory exercises like this one can be easier to perform. Questions About the Overload Principle In order to increase athletic performance and fitness, overloading is necessary. This strategy does, however, raise some serious questions about what can occur if you don't use it at all as well as what might occur if you use it incorrectly. Ignoring the Principle of Overload and Reaching a Stall Neglecting the overload principle seems to have the drawback of not producing gains. You can only make so much progress if you continue to train at the same frequency and intensity.

After that, you are at a plateau with no further increases or adaptations and are not straining the muscles any more. This happens as a result of how well our bodies handle stress. Your novice customer is initially rather concerned by that five-pound weight. The client feels stronger right away. Five-pound weights are no longer adequate, though, as the amount of stress needed to develop new responses grows with time. Excessive training and attainment However, you run the risk of overreaching or overtraining if you apply the overload principle wrong, for as by increasing intensity too fast.

Overreaching is a transient problem that results in a decline in physical performance from which one must recover over several days. An extended period of high training stress is called overtraining. Weeks or months may pass before performance returns to normal at this point. The following are signs of overtraining that you should be aware of: The heart rate at rest has gone up. Blood pressure is now higher. Loss of appetite and weight issues with sleeping. Changes in emotions or moods. Weary. A persistent aching in the muscles. There are longer recovery times. Overloading Techniques and Approaches Here are some guidelines to follow if you're just starting to use progressive overload with your clients: Try to develop gradually. The risk of injury increases when a client's workout volume is increased too quickly. Overusing a muscle can happen easily. Therefore, aim for small steps. If they are currently using a 5-pound weight, increase it to 7 pounds. Raise it to 10 to 12 if their rep count is between 8 and 10. Reduce your speed to prevent overusing or overstretching the muscle. Remember the goals of the client. Everybody approaches increasing overload in a different way. They should increase the weight used, lower the number of reps, and extend the rest period in between sets if they want to get stronger. In the event when building muscle is the goal, a heavier weight would be required. On the other hand, the number of reps would rise instead of fall, and the amount of time spent recovering would also fall instead of rising. They could desire physical stamina.

This means doing more repetitions with a lower weight. Make modifications to the instruction in just one area at a time. After the client has done gaining, increase the weight utilized, add another resistance training session to the week, or make another modification. Avoid making all of these adjustments at once. Just one at a time, please. Once they're familiar with one phase, change something else. There are a lot of ways to make sure your customer doesn't become overstimulated or hit a wall. All of these strategies basically involve making an activity better in some way. Together, these many elements create the FITT principle, or frequency. The number of times per week that your customer works out is typically measured. Increasing frequency can, for instance, mean going from one to two lifting sessions per week.

vigor. This is how hard your customer is working in a training session. By using heavier weights during strength training, you can intensify the workout. One useful method for determining the intensity of aerobic exercise is heart rate measurement. Momentum. When you progress and overload at an activity, like lifting or running, you may have to put in more time to do it. Sort of. The type is specific to the exercise that your client is performing. For example, you can change the type of strength training such that it targets a different muscle or muscle group. For instance, mix leg pushes and squats to strain the leg muscles. Changing the variables that you tweak for your clients is essential. One day, for instance, you might focus on using heavier weights to increase intensity. In the following session, try switching up your focus and spending more time with weights. For aerobic adaptations, a runner might, for instance, concentrate on heart rate or interval training one day to build intensity, and then the next week, extend the time with a long, leisurely run. Changing up the way you overload your body could help lower the chance that your progress will plateau. Putting too much on Recommendations for Gradual and Safe Overloading Overloading need to be incremental and gradual at all times. Increasing training volume, frequency, repetitions, and other factors too quickly might be dangerous. Injuries, sore muscles, and, of course, overtraining are possible outcomes.

Use these tips to keep overload progressive and safe for your clients: It is imperative that advancements are made gradually. A five-pound bicep curl cannot be increased to a twenty-pound bicep curl without running the danger of harm, overreaching, or overtraining. Develop a deliberate plan for escalating training components one by one. Prior to raising the weight for strength training, focus on form. Increasing time and frequency before stepping up the intensity is a good way to get better at lifting weights. Increase the weight progressively for more intensity after your client has mastered a particular exercise in safe, outstanding form. Test your client's maximums to determine appropriate weight levels and intensity increases. Monitoring your workouts and how you're upping the frequency, intensity, length, and kind is also a smart idea. Allocate time for relaxation. At this point, development occurs and overtraining and injuries are avoided. Recovery can take the form of alternate days of easy and hard workouts or an active rest day with a light activity, such taking a stroll. Keep your customer from growing weary of instruction.

It's never a good idea to exercise until you pass out or become exhausted because this will most likely result in overtraining. Three Instances of the Progressive Overload Theory Case Studies How does using progressive overload affect a resistance training program? Think about the following examples: Example No. 1: Weight Gain Advancement Right now, your client is extending his triceps by 60 pounds. For a few weeks, raise the weight to 65 pounds to aid in their improvement. Once that seems comfortable, increase the weight to seventy pounds. Maintain the 5-pound weight increase schedule, adding weight every 3.4–5 weeks. Example #2: Advancement through Rep Raising On lower body days, you typically have your client execute eight to ten squats. Up the rep count to ten or twelve. Next, raise it to 12 or 15. When they reach the necessary number of repetitions, you can start escalating their sets. Just remember not to increase their sets and reps at the same time. Lower their rep count as soon as you start increasing their sets. By doing this, you can prevent overusing the muscle.

Example #3: Increases in Training Session Progression If the customer's training has reached a standstill, extend the session. Have them work out for 50 minutes as opposed to 45 minutes. Increase this duration by 55 minutes and then by an hour. Every week, you also raise the quantity of completed sessions. Up the number of times you train each week from two to three. From three to four trainers, increase the number. (If they work out with weights four days a week, make sure to schedule their program to allow adequate recovery time for the muscle regions you work.) One strategy to prevent overloading-related overtraining is periodization. You can use periodization in the workouts that your client performs. Your client shouldn't go in a linear fashion in order to get the benefits of overloading. It is not a good idea to make each exercise harder, faster, or longer than the last one. Training periodization implies that variance need to be higher. Periodization is the exact way that training cycles are arranged. It is a crucial training strategy to support the overload idea. You have to switch up your workouts to overload your body in order to get better and see results.

But you also need to take into account the general adaptation syndrome (GAS) theory, which says that high-intensity training needs to be followed by low-intensity training or rest. By periodizing your training with cycles of longer, more intensive sessions and cycles of lower intensity for rest and recovery, you may prepare for higher overload. Three different types of cycles are included in a periodized training plan: Large-scale cycles. The macrocycle is an extended training session that might extend from half a year to a full year. The macrocycle might culminate in a single event, like a fitness competition, or it can correlate with a sports season, like running competitions in the summer and fall. Your client will have big, overarching macrocycle goals, like reaching a certain time goal for finishing a marathon. Mesocycles. Three to four mesocycles, each lasting a few weeks to a month, make up a macrocycle.

You may use these cycles to accomplish smaller goals, like running a 10k and then a half marathon. They might focus on particular training elements, like lifting weight or hypertrophy. tiny cycles. These shorter cycles last one to two weeks, at most. Every microcycle is a representation of the particular exercises you create for your client while maintaining the main goals and points of emphasis. By using periodization, you can modify your client's entire training regimen and take advantage of overload by incorporating low-intensity or appropriate rest periods. In order to accomplish the overall macrocycle objectives, it is necessary to alter the emphasis of each mesocycle and the varied sessions within each microcycle in order to provide enough overload, variation, and recovery time. A key idea in fitness is the overload principle. If you do not put the body under stress, you will never see improvements in physical strength, endurance, size, or aerobic fitness. Your body will overstress if you overtrain, which can lower your performance or possibly cause an injury. Achieving the right balance is essential for progress that is steady and slow.

Additionally, you may help your clients overload in the right way when combined with periodization in a well-designed training program, leading to notable improvements in fitness as well as the accomplishment of performance and sports goals.